Platelets in Cardiovascular Disease

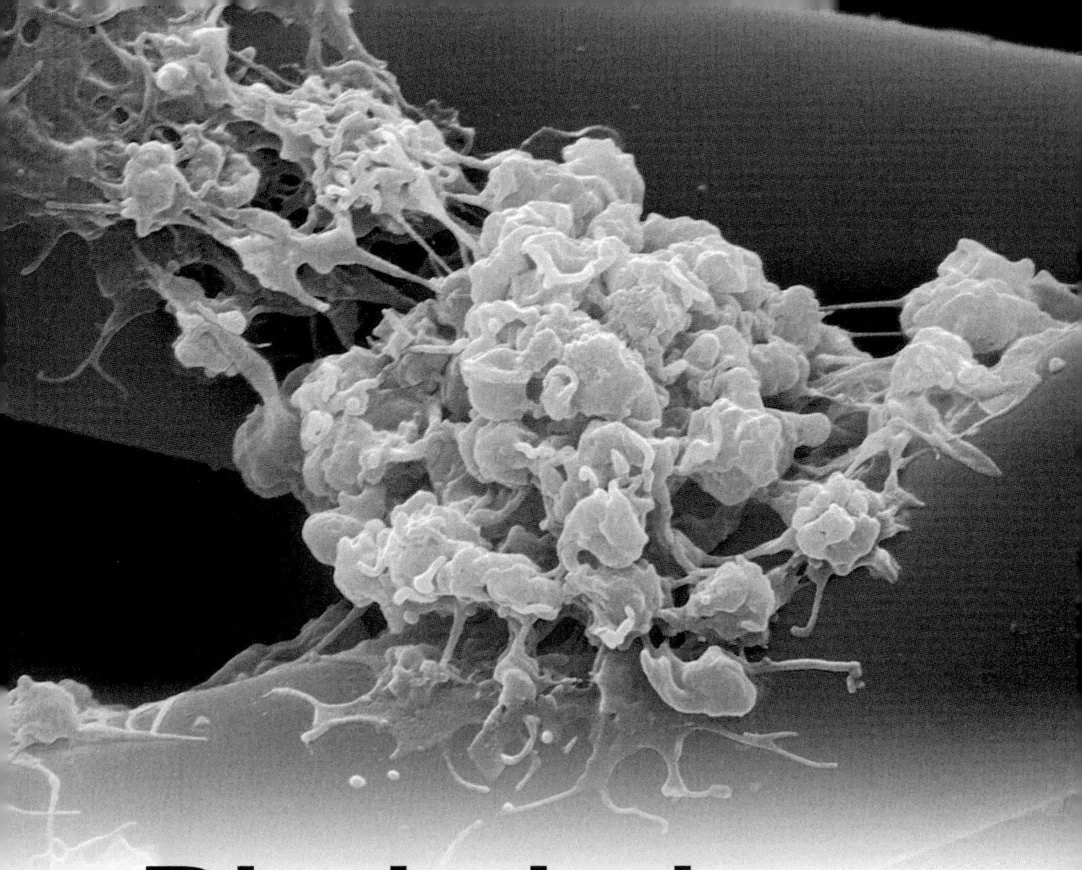

Platelets in Cardiovascular Disease

Editor

Deepak L. Bhatt
Cleveland Clinic, USA

ICP
Imperial College Press

Published by

Imperial College Press
57 Shelton Street
Covent Garden
London WC2H 9HE

Distributed by

World Scientific Publishing Co. Pte. Ltd.
5 Toh Tuck Link, Singapore 596224
USA office: 27 Warren Street, Suite 401-402, Hackensack, NJ 07601
UK office: 57 Shelton Street, Covent Garden, London WC2H 9HE

British Library Cataloguing-in-Publication Data
A catalogue record for this book is available from the British Library.

PLATELETS IN CARDIOVASCULAR DISEASE

ISBN-13 978-1-86094-826-8
ISBN-10 1-86094-826-X

Typeset by Stallion Press
Email: enquiries@stallionpress.com

Printed in Singapore by Mainland Press Pte Ltd

To my wife Shanthala and to my sons Vinayak,
Arjun, and Ram, for their support,
encouragement, and understanding
of my passion for platelets!

Contents

Contributors

Richard C. Becker, MD
Divisions of Cardiovascular Medicine and Hematology
Duke University School of Medicine
Director
Duke Cardiovascular Thrombosis Center
Duke University Medical Center
Duke Clinical Research Institute
2400 Pratt Street
Durham, NC 27705, USA

Christopher P. Cannon, MD
Senior Investigator, TIMI Study
350 Longwood Ave, 1st Floor
Boston, MA 02115, USA
Associate Physician, Cardiovascular Division
Brigham and Women's Hospital
75 Francis Street
Boston, MA 02115, USA
Associate Professor of Medicine
Harvard Medical School

Derek P. Chew, MBBS, MPH, FRACP
Associate Professor of Medicine
Flinders University
Interventional Cardiologist
Director of Acute Coronary Syndrome Programs
and Cardiovascular Outcomes Research
Department of Cardiovascular Medicine
Flinders Medical Center
Flinders Drive, Bedford Park
South Australia, 5042, Australia

Brian R. Dulin, MD
Department of Internal Medicine
University of Kentucky
900 S. Limestone Avenue
326 Charles T. Wethington Bldg.
Lexington, KY 40536-0200, USA

Robert A. Harrington, MD, FACC, FAHA, FSCAI
Professor, Division of Cardiology
Department of Medicine, Duke University Medical Center
Director, Duke Clinical Research Institute
7007 North Pavilion, 2400 Pratt Street
Durham, NC 27705, USA

Paul Harrison, BSc, PhD, MRCPath
Clinical Scientist and Honorary Lecturer
Oxford Haemophilia Center and Thrombosis Unit
Churchill Hospital, Oxford, OX3 7LJ, UK

Brian K. Jefferson, MD
Fellow
Department of Interventional Cardiology
Cleveland Clinic Foundation
9500 Euclid Avenue
Cleveland, OH 44195, USA

Juhana Karha, MD
Fellow in Interventional Cardiology
Department of Cardiovascular Medicine
Cleveland Clinic Foundation
9500 Euclid Avenue
Cleveland, OH 44195, USA

Kandice Kottke-Marchant, MD, PhD
Chair, Division of Pathology and Laboratory Medicine
Department of Pathology and Laboratory Medicine
Cleveland Clinic Foundation
9500 Euclid Ave. / L21
Cleveland, OH 44195, USA

Sam J. Lehman, MBBS
Cardiology Fellow
Flinders University
Department of Cardiovascular Medicine
Flinders Medical Center
Flinders Drive, Bedford Park
South Australia, 5042, Australia

Alan D. Michelson, MD
Director, Center for Platelet Function Studies
Professor of Pediatrics, Medicine, and Pathology
University of Massachusetts Medical School
55 Lake Avenue North
Worcester, MA 01655, USA

Steven R. Steinhubl, MD
Director of CV Education and Clinical Research
Associate Professor of Medicine
Division of Cardiology
University of Kentucky
900 S. Limestone Avenue
326 Charles T. Wethington Bldg.
Lexington, KY 40536-0200, USA

Eric J. Topol, MD
Director, Scripps Translational Science Institute
Scripps Research Institute
10550 N. Torrey Pines Rd. MEM-275
La Jolla, CA 92037, USA

Harvey D. White, DSc
Green Lane Cardiovascular Service
Auckland City Hospital
Private Bag 92024
Auckland 1030, New Zealand

Preface

In medical school, I had learned that platelets were just passive participants in blood clot formation; other more important constituents of blood were the really key players in thrombosis and platelets were just "along for the ride." As the science of platelets evolved, it became clear that platelets were active mediators of thrombus formation, central in the pathogenesis of acute ischemic syndromes, including heart attacks and strokes.

More recently, the roles of platelets as immune cells and active biosynthetic factories, churning out all sorts of biological mediators, have become evident. Thus, the platelet has morphed into a truly critical part of cardiovascular medicine, as have therapies directed toward inhibiting platelet function.

I am extremely grateful to the chapter authors of this book, experts in not only the science of platelets, but also in clinical cardiovascular care. They have summarized the key aspects of platelet biology and anti-platelet therapies in a manner that should be of great interest and practical utility to health care providers as well as scientists in the field. I am also thankful to the Imperial College Press for their guidance in preparing what I hope readers will discover to be an exciting view of the past, present, and future of platelets and anti-platelet therapy.

Deepak L. Bhatt
MD, FACC, FSCAI, FESC, FACP

1 Platelet Biology
The Role of Platelets in Hemostasis, Thrombosis and Inflammation

Richard C. Becker

Introduction

Platelets, much more than a passive, circulating, anuclear cellular element, play a vital role in physiologic hemostasis by stemming blood loss and initiating tissue healing in response to vascular trauma. Similar, yet biologically amplified processes place the platelet centrally in the natural history and phenotypic expression of atherothrombotic vascular disease.

The following chapter summarizes the structural-functional characteristics of platelet biology and emphasizes the importance of cell-cell interactions, cellular surface events, intracellular protein signaling and fundamental biochemistry toward achieving safe, effective and targeted therapeutics.

Platelet: Structural Anatomy

Simple in appearance, the platelet is functionally complex. The structure-function is best understood by dividing the resting platelet into four anatomically distinct zones.[1]

Peripheral zone

The peripherial zone consists of a membrane and its invaginations, which form the open canalicular system. It can be divided into three distinct domains: the exterior coat, the unit membrane, and the submembrane region.

Exterior coat

The exterior COAT is 10–20 nm thick glycocalyx and rich in glycoproteins.[2–5] A majority serve as receptors for cell-cell and cell-vessel wall interactions. They are discussed in greater detail within the sections to follow on platelet adhesion and aggregation.

Platelet unit membrane

The platelet unit membrane is similar to other blood cell membranes in several ways: (1) it consists of a lipid bilayer rich in phospholipids; (2) it provides a physiochemical separation between intracellular and extracellular processes; and (3) it contains anion and cation pumps (i.e. Na^+/K^+-ATPase) critical to the maintenance of transmembrane ionic gradients. The platelet membrane is an important catalyst for fluid-phase coagulation.[6,7]

Submembrane region

The area beneath the unit membrane is appropriately called the *submembrane region*. It contains a distinct network of microfilaments that are anatomically (and functionally) associated with both membrane glycoproteins and an extensive cytoplasmic filament system.[8,9]

Sol-gel zone

The matrix of the cytoplasm is called the *sol-gel zone* and consists of two fiber systems in varying states of polymerization. Just beneath the submembrane region are tightly coiled microtubules that help maintain resting platelet shape.[10] With activation the microtubules constrict into tight rings around centrally clustered organelles. The driving force for this contractile event is actually provided by the cytoplasmic filaments (not the microtubules).

The second set of fibers within the sol-gel zone are the actin microfilaments. In the resting platelet only 30%–40% of actin is polymerized into filaments.[11] With activation there is an increase in polymerization, with new filaments appearing at the cell periphery and within developing filopedia.[12]

Organelle zone

The organelle zone is not, in the purest sense, a distinct zone but contains storage granules, dense bodies, peroxisomes, lysosomes, and mitochondria dispersed throughout the cytoplasm. As such this zone is centrally involved with metabolic processes and also acts as a storage site for enzymes, adenine nucleotides, serotonin, calcium, and a wide variety of proteins.

Membrane system

The membrane system constitutes the fourth and final zone. The plasma membrane also contains numerous invaginations that course deep within the platelet. Commonly referred to as the *open canalicular system*, these channels provide a large surface area for cellular transport and remain patent (and functionally active) throughout platelet activation, with shape change, and during the release reaction.[13,14]

The dense tubular system represents a second membrane system located within the cell's interior. Derived from parent cell endoplasmic reticulum, the dense tubular system acts as a storage site for calcium as well as for the enzymes involved in prostaglandin synthesis.[15,16] The two membrane systems are in direct communication with one another, allowing for an exchange of contents.

Platelet: Functional Anatomy

Under normal conditions, platelets circulate freely in blood vessels without interacting with other platelets or the vascular endothelium. In the presence of endothelial damage, whether from vascular injury or rupture of an atherosclerotic plaque, a chain of events is triggered, leading to platelet-rich clot formation. Depending on the initiating event, this may represent normal hemostasis or pathologic vascular thrombosis. The responsible events represent a complex series of biochemical and cellular processes that can be loosely divided into four general categories: adhesion, activation, secretion and aggregation.[17]

Platelet adhesion

Platelets adhere avidly to damaged, disrupted or dysfunctional vascular endothelium. This is especially true in areas of exposed subendothelial collagen and lipid deposits, as found in eroded or ruptured atherosclerotic plaques. Coverage of the exposed site by platelets is mediated by adhesive proteins that are recognized by specific platelet membrane glycoproteins. These glycoproteins are also critical for cell-cell interactions.

To date nine of the predominant platelet membrane glycoproteins have been characterized.[2–5] The most common nomenclature for identification is based on polyacrylamide gel separation. With increasing sophistication of the gel systems, increasing separation within groups has been achieved.

Most platelet membrane receptors consist of non-covalent complexes of individual glycoproteins. The various surface membrane glycoproteins and their ligands are summarized in Table 1. There is considerable functional overlap as several receptors may bind the same ligand and a specific receptor may response to more than one ligand. The receptors can also be divided into integrins and non-integrins. Integrins are heterodimeric cell-surface

Table 1. Surface membrane glycoprotein receptors.

Receptor	Ligand	Integrin components	Biologic action
GPIa/IIa	Collagen	$\alpha_2\beta_1$	Adhesion
GPIb/IX	von Willebrand factor	–	Adhesion
GPIc/IIa	Fibronectin	$\alpha_5\beta_1$	Adhesion
GPIIb/IIIa	Collagen Fibrinogen Fibronectin Vitronectin von Willebrand factor	$\alpha_{IIb}\beta_3$	Aggregation (secondary role in adhesion)
GPIV	Thrombospondin, collagen	–	Adhesion
GPVI	Collagen		
Vitronectin receptor	Vitronectin Thrombospondin	$A_v\beta_3$	Adhesion
VLA-6	Laminin	$A_6\beta_1$	Adhesion

molecules composed of α- and β-subunits. Platelets express at least two β-subunits (β_1 and β_2) and five α-subunits, which in varying combination identify distinct surface receptors.[18]

The initiating event for adhesion is contact, a process during which an inactivated circulating platelet "stops" and "sticks" to a site of vascular damage.[19] This important event is accomplished by an interaction between the platelet glycoprotein Ib-IX complex and von Willebrand (vWF), a large protein synthesized by vascular endothelial cells and secreted on both the luminal and subendothelial surfaces. vWF also has functional domains that contribute to the binding of platelets to vessel wall constituents (collagen, microfibrils).[20,21]

A unique feature of platelet adhesion is its dependence on shearing forces. In fact, without forces of at least 600–3000 A^{-1} between surfaces, platelet "contact" will not occur.[22–24] Adhesion of platelets to vascular subendothelial components represents the primary hemostatic response to vessel wall injury. It also effects a strong stimulus for platelet activation via pathways mediated by the membrane glycoprotein receptors (outside-in signaling).

Platelet activation

Platelet activation can be triggered by a wide variety of biochemical and mechanical stimuli (in addition to platelet adhesion; Table 2). Many of the biochemical agonists are produced or released by platelets themselves after vessel wall adhesion, initiating a biological feedback loop that amplifies the response to a given stimulus.

Platelet agonists bind surface glycoprotein receptors and stimulate signal transduction across the membrane via messenger proteins (G-coupled) that, in turn, triggers one of two intracellular pathways. The phosphoinositide pathway is initiated with activation of phospholipase C. Phosphatidylinositol-4-5-biphosphate (PIP_2) is cleaved to form two secondary messengers, inositol-1,4,5-triphosphate (IP_3) and diacylglycerol.[25] IP_3 stimulates calcium mobilization from the dense tubular system, which in turn is required for activation of other intracellular enzymes responsible for physiologic platelet responses.[26] Diacylglycerol activates phospholipase C, causing protein phosphorylation, granule secretion, and fibrinogen receptor expression.

Table 2. Platelet structural and functional response to activation.

- Shape change and pseudopod formation
- Change in the conformation of GPIIb/IIIa to the form that binds fibrinogen and von Willebrand factor (ligand receptive)
- Increase in cytosolic Ca^{2+} due to influx from the exterior
- Cytoskeletal assembly
- Aggregation
- Activation of phospholipase C, producing the second messengers inositol-1,4,5-triphosphate (IP_3) and diacylglycerol
- Mobilization of Ca^{2+} from internal stores by IP_3
- Activation of phospholipase A2, leading to formation of thromboxane A2
- Activation of protein kinase C by diacylglycerol, leading to phosphorylation of a 47-kd protein
- Secretion of contents of α and dense granules (lysosomal granule contents secreted only upon strong stimulation)
- Surface expression of several α-granule proteins (e.g. thrombospondin and fibrinogen)
- Surface expression of granule membrane proteins (e.g. P-selectin)
- Development of coagulation activity by transbilayer movement of procoagulant phospholipids
- Inhibition of adenylyl cyclase
- Dephosphorylation of VASP — vasodilator-stimulated phosphoprotein
- Clot retraction

The second pathway involves phospholipase A_2, which following activation, liberates arachidonate from cell membranes. Arachidonate is subsequently converted to thromboxane A_2 (TxA_2) by the platelet's cycloxygenase enzyme system. TxA_2 is a potent platelet agonist in its own right, thus providing yet another positive feedback mechanism that promotes platelet-mediated thrombosis.

Platelet agonists can be classified (Table 3). Thrombin affects both phosphoinositide hydrolysis *and* arachidonate metabolism (via phospholipase C and phospholipase A_2). Accordingly, its ability to promote platelet activation and aggregation persists despite inhibition of one of the two pathways. Indeed, it has been shown that even low concentrations of thrombin (≤ 0.1 IU/mL) can produce platelet aggregation in the face of inhibition of platelet TxA_2 production.[27]

Table 3. Physiologic agonists for platelet activation.

Agonist	Source	Receptor(s)
Thrombin	End-product of coagulation cascade	PAR-1, PAR-4 GPIbα
Adenosine diphosphate (ADP)	Platelet dense body	$P2Y_1$, $P2Y_{12}$
Collagen	Subendothelium component	GPIa/IIa, GPIIb/IIIa, GPIV, GPVI
Serotonin	Platelet dense body	$5HT_2$ receptor
Thromboxane A_2	Produced by other cells	PGH_2, TXA_2 receptor
Platelet activating factor	Lipid mediator produced by other cells	PAF receptor

COAT platelets

Concomitant activation of platelets with two agonists, collagen and thrombin, yields a population of cells known as COAT platelets (collagen and thrombin activated) that are enriched in several membrane-bound, procoagulant proteins, including thrombospondin, factor V, fibronectin, fibrinogen and von Willebrand Factor.[28] Although the hemostatic function and contributing role of COAT platelets to atherothrombosis[29] is under active investigation, preliminary work suggests that they may be resistant to GPIIb/IIIa antagonists[30] — an observation of potential clinical relevance if confirmed.

Variability in platelet procoagulant potential observed *in vivo* suggests that, in contrast to the traditional paradigm of platelets either being "unactivated" or "activated," they may exist in several differing states of activation. It follows that a possible target for therapeutic intervention is the prevention (or modulation) of platelets, preventing highly activated (and procoagulant) states.

Two separate thrombin receptors have been identified on the platelet surface — a high-affinity receptor and a moderate-affinity receptor.[31,32] The high-affinity receptor is GPIbα. Observations that Bernard-Soulier platelets (congenitally deficient in GPIbα) are poorly activated by low levels of thrombin support this hypothesis.[33] Experiments in which GPIbα is cleaved also reveal an impaired response of platelets to lower (but not higher) concentrations of α-thrombin.[34,35]

The "moderate-affinity" receptor, known as the *thrombin receptor*, was first cloned by Coughlin and colleagues in 1991.[36] This receptor is a member of a G-protein-linked, seven transmembrane domain receptor family and is found on platelets, endothelial cells, smooth muscle cells and fibroblasts (Fig. 1). Thrombin interacts with at least two sites on this receptor's lengthy extracellular amino-terminal end. Thrombin cleaves the amino-terminal extension (at Arg^{41}-Ser^{42}) to expose a new amino terminus, that, in turn, acts as a "tethered ligand," which activates platelets by binding to an as yet unidentified region of the same receptor.[36–38]

Protease activated receptors (PAR), glycoprotein-coupled members of the seven transmembrane domain receptor super-family, are characterized by their ability to serve as specific substrates for regulatory proteases, which subsequently cleave one peptide bond in the molecule's extracellular domain. A new N-terminus of the receptor interacts with a separate domain of the cleaved receptor, causing its activation. PAR-1, -3, and -4 are predominantly thrombin receptors. PAR-2 is activated by trypsin, fXa, and fVIIa.[39–41]

PAR receptors have been detected and localized on vascular endothelial cells, mononuclear cells, platelets, fibroblasts, and smooth muscle cells. The expression of PAR-1 on platelets, endothelial cells, and atherosclerotic

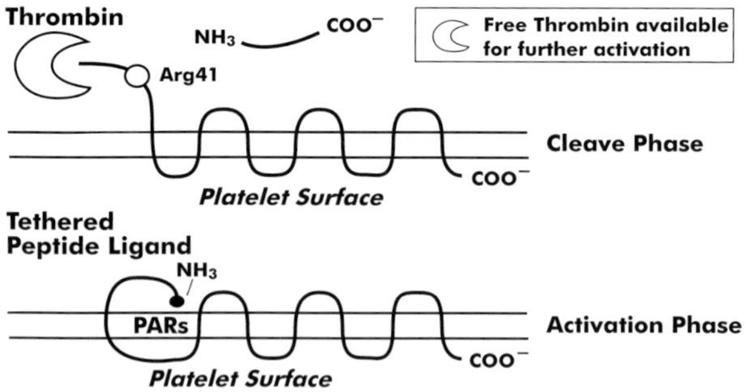

Fig. 1. Thrombin binds to its platelet receptor along a lengthy extracellular amino terminal extension. Thrombin cleaves the receptor at a specific site and exposes a new amino terminus, which then functions as a tethered peptide ligand to activate a receptor referred to as protease-activated receptors or PARs.

plaques supports its role in tissue response to injury, inflammation, and thrombosis. Activation of PAR-1 in endothelial cells induces expression of ICAM-1, VCAM-1, P-selectin, E-selectin, IL-6, IL-8, and a wide variety of growth factors.[42,43] A similar response is observed following PAR-2 activation, but in addition, it leads to von Willebrand factor release, tissue factor expression, and suppression of tissue factor pathway inhibitor.[44,45] The activation of PAR-1 in mast cells provokes histamine, platelet activating factor, and cytokine release.[46–48]

Platelet PAR-1 and PAR-4 activation initiates several glycoprotein-coupled signaling pathways, including G_q, $G_{12/13}$, G_i, and G_2, which in turn provoke platelet shape change, dense granule release, thromboxane A_2 generation, glycoprotein IIb/IIIa activation, and procoagulant responses (prothrombinase activity and thrombin generation). While platelet release and aggregation can occur following activation of either PAR-1 or PAR-4, procoagulant activity requires complimentary activation of both receptors.[49,50]

Platelet secretion

Platelet activation, a complex response to extracellular signals, prompts cytoskeleton rearrangements, membrane fusion, exteriorization and secretion (exocytosis) of contents from within three different types of platelet storage granules: lysosomes, α-granules, and dense bodies. Fusion of α-granules with each other and with deep invaginations of the plasma membrane (the open canalicular system) followed by an "emptying" of contents to the exterior has been demonstrated.[51,52]

The lysosomes contain a number of acid hydrolases (cathepsins) that digest endocytosed materials. Lysosome secretion occurs more slowly than does dense granule or α-granule secretion.[53–55]

The platelet also contains a small number of osmophylic electron-dense granules, referred to as *dense bodies* (or dense core). They contain a large amount of non-metabolic adenines (ADP, GDP), as well as divalent cations (Ca^{2+}, Mg^{2+}), serotonin, and pyrophosphates. ADP secretion following platelet activation promotes recruitment and activation of additional platelets to the site of vascular injury.

The platelet α-granules are spherical (300–500 nm in diameter) bodies, each with an eccentric staining pattern. They contain platelet-specific proteins, coagulation factors, and a variety of glycoproteins. Among the platelet-specific proteins are several peptides that modulate cell growth. Of these, platelet-derived growth factor (PDGF) is among the most extensively studied. Two distinct receptors for PDGF have been isolated on smooth muscle cells and fibroblasts.[56] It has been suggested that PDGF modulates smooth muscle cell proliferation that occurs following platelet-vessel wall interaction. Two other structurally related α-granule proteins are connecting tissue activating peptide III (CTAP III) and platelet factor-4. CTAP III is involved with fibroblast proliferation and represents a precursor to β-thromboglobulin.[57] Platelet factor-4 binds to heparin and effectively neutralizes its anticoagulant activity. It also participates in inflammatory reactions through chemotactic effects on neutrophils and monocytes.[58]

Platelet α-granules contain a number of coagulation proteins. Of physiologic importance, 20%–25% of blood factor V is stored within platelet α-granules, and it has been demonstrated that platelet factor V is the major protein secreted and phosphorylated following α-thrombin stimulation.[59,60] Accordingly, platelet factor V is critical to the assembly of prothrombinase, which can then generate additional thrombin. Platelets also contain protein S (the cofactor for protein C-mediated factor V and VIII inhibition). It has been postulated that protein C may exert is anticoagulant effect largely at sites of platelet adhesion and activation.[61] Release of plasminogen activator inhibitor-1 (PAI-1) plays a contributing role in modulating local fibrinolytic potential.[62] Platelets also contain and release fibrinogen. Although meager in comparison with plasma levels, platelet fibrinogen is more highly concentrated, suggesting further that platelets provide a site for localizing hemostatic responses.[63]

Platelet α-granules contains at least seven different glycoproteins; some are secreted, while others bind to the granule membrane. The major soluble glycoprotein secreted is thrombospondin. Also secreted by endothelial cells, thrombospondin is thought to play a role in the regulation of smooth muscle cell proliferation.[64] There is also an internal storage pool of GP IIb/IIIa within the α-granules. Following activation they are expressed on the platelet surface and can increase the total number of surface GPIIb/IIIa receptors by up to twofold.[65–67]

The platelet ADP receptor

Adenosine diphosphate (ADP) was the first nucleotide identified in blood that could account for changes in platelet behavior upon exposure to a foreign surface. In fact, ADP extracted from erythrocyte membranes was shown to increase the ability of platelets to stick to glass,[68,69] an effect that was subsequently shown to require calcium and fibrinogen. Since that time, a wide variety of pharmacological responses to nucleotides have been identified, fostering the creation of comprehensive classification of nucleotide receptors.[70–72]

Purinergic receptors are cell surface receptors that selectively bind ATP or ADP over adenosine. The surface receptors for extracellular nucleotides are referred to as P2 receptors, whereas P1 purinoreceptors preferentially recognize adenosine. The present day nomenclature for P2 receptors is based on molecular structure and signal transduction mechanisms. Accordingly, P2X receptors are ligand-gated ion channels, while P2Y receptors are G-protein coupled. $P2Y_1$ and $P2Y_{12}$ are both activated by ADP. Once activated, $P2Y_1$ activates phospholipase C and triggers shape change, while $P2Y_{12}$ couples to Gi, reducing adenylyl cyclase activity. Functionally, $P2Y_1$ receptor activation initiates platelet aggregation, but $P2Y_{12}$ is required for full platelet aggregation and stabilization in response to ADP.

Binding

The binding of [^{14}C] ADP to the platelet surface is achieved through a specific receptor site (molecular weight, 61 kDa) with approximately 100,000 copies per cell (affinity constant $K = 6.5 \times 10^6 M^{-1}$.[73] Competition for binding of [^{3}H]-ADP is as follows: ATP = ADP > adenosine monophosphate (AMP) $\gg$ adenosine.

Mechanisms of action

A variety of platelet responses have been reported following the binding of ADP to its receptor, including rapid calcium influx, mobilization of intracellular calcium stores, shape change, inhibition of adenylyl cyclase, stimulation of IP_3 formation, expression of surface GPIIb/IIIa, stimulation of phospholipase A_2, release of dense granules contents, and release of α-granule contents.

The important contributions of ADP and its platelet receptor to vascular hemostasis and pathological thrombosis are supported by the observed bleeding tendencies among individuals with inherited abnormalities in ADP binding and ADP-mediated platelet aggregation.[74,75]

ADP accelerates and potentiates tissue factor-induced thrombin generation via stimulation of $P2Y_{12}$ receptors. This particular receptor also mediates the potentiating effect of PAR-1 stimulation on thrombin generation and is paralleled by surface phosphatidyl serine exposure.[76]

ADP receptors on other cells

ADP receptors exist on cells other than platelets and may have physiological importance. ADP promotes the binding of fibrinogen to monocytes[77] and stimulates calcium mobilization in megakarocytes. ADP receptors have also been identified on glioma cells, hepatocytes, and capillary endothelial cells.[78]

Platelet aggregation

An important platelet response which follows platelet activation is a conformational change in the membrane receptor GPIIb/IIIa. This allows fibrinogen and the GPIIb/IIIa receptor to interact, forming multiple crosslinks between adjacent platelets.

GPIIb/IIIa is a member of the integrin family of receptors, composed of α- and β-subunits (α_{IIb}, β_3). The α-subunit consists of a heavy chain and a light chain. The heavy chain is entirely extracellular, while the light chain spans the platelet membrane, ending in a short extracellular domain.[79]

With platelet activation, GPIIb/IIIa undergoes a conformational change, rendering it competent to bind protein ligands in general and fibrinogen in particular. While the underlying biochemical mechanism for this transformation is not entirely clear, electron microscopy studies of the GPIIb/IIIa-fibrinogen complex have provided several important insights.[80] The globular head of GPIIb/IIIa interacts with the distal end of the fibrinogen molecule; the tails are extended laterally at an angle of 90° to the long axis of the fibrinogen molecule. Thus with GPIIb/IIIa binding toward opposite ends of a fibrinogen molecule, the tails are oriented to opposite sides, enabling a "bridge" to be formed between two adjacent platelets.

Cell-based model of coagulation

A revised "cell-based" model of coagulation [81] proposes that blood clotting occurs not as a cascade, but in three integrated and overlapping stages:

- initiation, which occurs on tissue factor-bearing cells;
- amplification or priming, in which platelets and cofactors are activated in preparation for large-scale thrombin generation; and
- propagation, during which there is a "burst" of thrombin generation (Fig. 2).

A cell-based model of coagulation provides a basis for other important cellular interactions among platelets, leukocytes and activated endothelial cells critical in the development and clinical expression of atherothrombosis (Fig. 3).[82] In addition, the construct provides an explanation for varying thrombotic potential between individuals through the identification of coagulation protein binding sites on the surface of activated platelets (Fig. 4).[83]

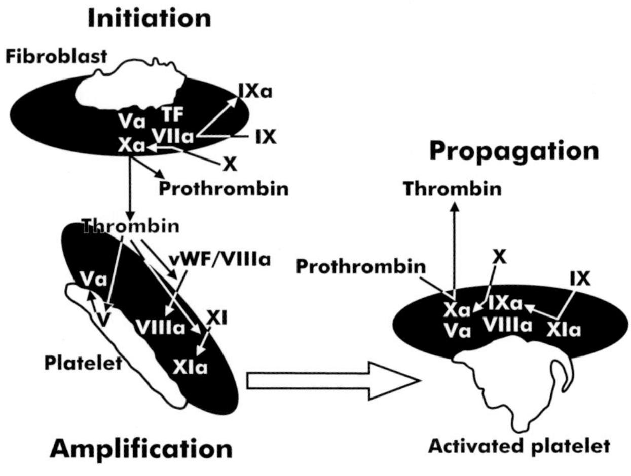

Fig. 2. The three phases of coagulation occur on different cell surfaces: initiation on the tissue factor-bearing cell; amplification on the platelet as it becomes activated; and propagation on the activated platelet surface. With permission from Hoffman M, A cell-based model of hemostasis, *Thromb Haemost* 2001;**85**:958–965.[81]

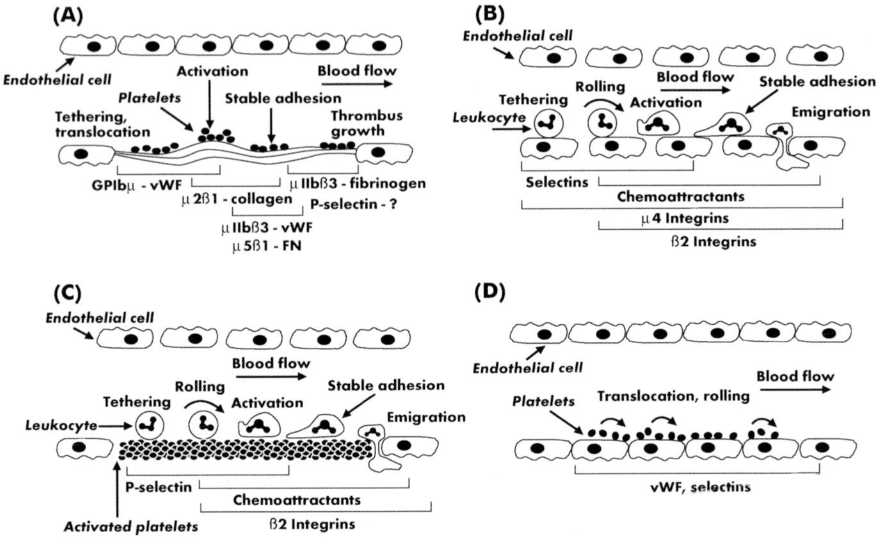

Fig. 3. (**A**) Adhesion of platelets to subendothelial surfaces. (**B**) Adhesion of leukocytes to activated endothelial cells. (**C**) Adhesion of leukocytes to activated platelets. (**D**) Adhesion of platelets to activated endothelial cells. With permission from McEver RP, Adhesive interactions of leukocytes, platelets, and the vessel wall during hemostasis and inflammation, *Thromb Haemost* 2001;**86**:746–756.[82]

Conceptually, the localization of coagulation to several cellular surfaces not only establishes an important mechanism for regulation but also expands the number of targets for therapeutic attenuation substantially.

Variability in aggregatory response to traditional platelet agonists may identify a group of "hyper-responders" in whom molecular and/or proteomic profiles and phenotypic characteristics could prove particularly useful for risk assessment and possibly management.[84]

Platelet-leukoctye interactions

Activated platelets release a wide variety of mediators that trigger and modulate inflammatory responses. There is evidence that platelets remain functional *in vivo* even after activation;[85,86] and when bound to damaged endothelium, still respond to agonist stimulation hours after adhesion has taken place.[87] Disaggregation of thrombi *in vitro* yields platelets that maintain basal morphology and secretory potential.[88] Similarly, platelets encased in a fibrin network express newly synthesized proinflammatory cytokines

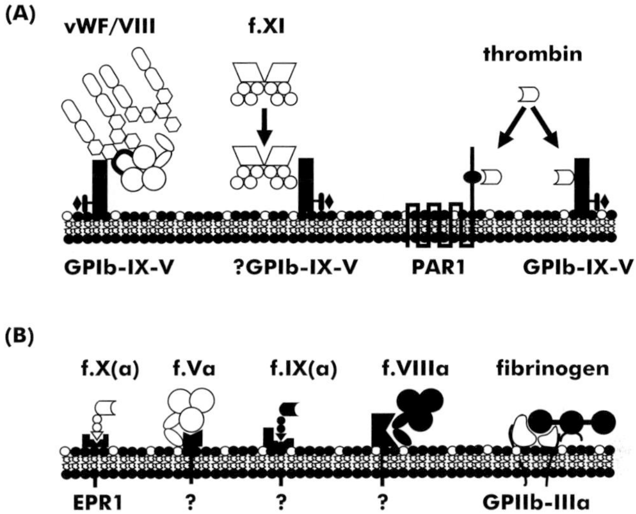

Fig. 4. Platelet binding proteins important in coagulation. Known platelet proteins are labeled below the protein. Proteins that have not yet been identified but that are suspected are indicated by question marks. Binding proteins thought to be important in the priming phase are shown in panel (**A**). Binding proteins thought to be important in the propagation phase are shown in panel (**B**). Activity associated with proteins in the propagation phase is not found on unactivated platelets, and activation appears to be required either for physical appearance of the protein on the outer leaflet of platelets or for activation of these proteins as in the case of GP IIb-IIIa. f.XI indicates factor XI; f.X(a), either factor X or factor Xa; f.Va, factor Va; f.IX(a), either factor IX or factor IXa; and f.VIIIa, factor VIIIa. With permission from Monroe DM, Platelets and thrombin generation, *Arterioscler Thromb Vasc Biol* 2002;**22**:1381–1389.[83]

for at least 18 hours after clot formation[89] and adhesion between platelets and leukocytes remains stable over time,[90–93] with gene expression in target leukocytes that increases steadily over the subsequent 24 hours.[92] Even platelets ingested by leukocytes modulate survival markers for days, suggesting the possibility that platelets can regulate inflammatory and perhaps thrombotic events both locally and systemically (at thrombosis-prone sites). Thrombin-stimulated platelets synthesize pro-IL-1β and augment its subsequent processing to a biologically active protein.[89] Circulating platelets then deliver this and other signaling proteins to target cells that amplify *in situ* inflammatory responses. For example, IL-1β triggers the synthesis of E-selectin, IL-8 and ENA-78 (required for leukocyte adhesion to endothelial cells). In addition, circulating platelet-leukocyte aggregates are stable and contribute to the "piggybacking" of platelets onto inflamed tissues during leukocyte transmigration.[93]

It could be stated that platelets are to thrombosis as leukocytes are to inflammation. However, over the past decade there has been increasing recognition that inflammation and thrombosis are linked intimately at several levels. Study of the modulating effects of neutrophils and platelets on one another became possible with improved methods for the preparation of platelet-free neutrophils and platelet-rich plasma.[94] Early studies focused on the ability of platelets or neutrophils to enhance each other's response to an aggregating stimulus. Reintroduction of platelets to a neutrophil preparation increased the neutrophil response to various chemotactic agents.[94,95] Similarly, reintroduction of activated neutrophils to a platelet preparation caused either direct platelet aggregation or increased the response to various agonists.[96–99]

Neutrophil-mediated cytoxicity, oxidant production, lysosome release and arachodonic acid metabolism are all increased in the presence of platelets.[7–9,94,100–104] Platelets activated by platelet activating factor have increased calcium mobilization and thromboxane β_2 release in the presence of activated neutrophils.[99] The capacity of platelets and leukocytes to modulate one another's activity is potentially explained by one or more mechanisms: (1) release of soluble mediators, (2) metabolism of released mediators, (3) presentation of surface-bound mediators, and (4) direct cell adhesion.

Platelet-derived mediators

The release of TxA_2 from activated platelets has been shown to enhance polymorphonulcear leukocytes (PMN) adhesiveness,[105] to mediate PMN diapedesis (via regulation of PMN adhesion receptor C18),[106] and to regulate the effect of activated neutrophils on atherosclerotic arterial vasoconstriction.[107,108] In turn, TxA_2 inhibition decreases neutrophil accumulation in ischemic myocardium with a subsequent reduction in experimental infarct size.[109–114] Platelet-derived growth factor (PDGF) induces PMN chemotaxis and stimulates phagocytosis;[115,116] however it also inhibits oxygen-derived free radical release from stimulated neutrophils. Plasma PDGF is decreased among patients with acute MI or unstable angina.[117] Other platelet-derived mediators shown to have effects on neutrophil

Table 4. Platelet-derived mediators influencing neutrophil function.

Platelet-derived mediator	Effect on neutrophil
TxA_2	Enhances PMN adhesiveness Mediates PMN diapedesis Regulates neutrophil effect on atherosclerotic vessel; Vasocontricts
PDGF	Induces PMN chemotaxis Stimulates PMN phagocytosis Inhibits activated PMN O_2-release
PF4	Induces PMN chemotaxis Stimulates PMN elastase release
12-HETE/12-HPETE	Induces PMN chemotaxis Stimulates PMN oxidative burst Promotes PMN adhesion to endothelium Modulates PMN stimulation with increased shear
Serotonin	Enhances PMN adherence to endothelium
Adenosine	May inhibit PMN activation

TxA_2 = Thromboxane A_2; PDGF = platelet-derived growth factor; PF-4 = platelet factor-4; PMN = polymorphonuclear leukocyte.
From Siminiak *et al.*[124] with permission.

function include platelet factor-4, 12-HETE/12-HPETE, and serotonin (Table 4).[106,115–124]

Neutrophil-derived mediators

Oxygen-derived free radicals, released by activated PMNs, can have either excitatory or inhibitory effects on platelets. Superoxide anion has been shown to act synergistically with thrombin to activate platelets and to stimulate serotonin release.[125] In contrast, there is at least one published report suggesting that PMN-derived H_20_2 can inhibit platelet aggregation.[126]

Elastases secreted from neutrophils have been found to inhibit thrombin-mediated platelet activation and serotonin release by cleaving specific platelet receptors.[127] Platelet-derived PF4 may stimulate the release of PMN elastase,[119] representing another potentially important link between platelets and PMNs.

Arachadonic acid metabolites derived from neutrophils may be utilized by platelets. For example, leukocyte-derived 5-HETE is the precursor for the platelet product 5,12-diHETE.[127] PMN-derived leukotrienes have been shown to enhance platelet aggregation in response to several agonists.[128] Finally, activated neutrophils can activate platelets by presenting surface-bound PAF.[129] This event requires cell-cell interaction and, in addition, may depend on direct adherence.

Platelet-leukocyte adhesion

Platelet-leukocyte adhesion is of physiologic importance for a variety of reasons. Close contact of cells ensures increased local concentrations of released mediators and provides a means of protection against circulating plasma inhibitors. Indeed, it has been shown that platelet activation by neutrophil-derived mediators is augmented if neutrophils are present within the *in vitro* preparation.[96,99] Adhesion between platelets and neutrophils itself may provide a stimulus for subsequent intracellular signaling events.

It is well documented that neutrophils and platelets bind to regions of vessel wall damage. While they clearly interact, independent function is often required of each. Thrombocytopenia is not, in and of itself, associated with an impaired immune response, nor is neutropenia linked with hemostatic abnormalities. Although the interaction between neutrophils and platelets may not be essential for normal physiologic function, it may play a role in the pathologic thrombosis, reperfusion injury, and chronic inflammation.[130]

The *in vitro* adherence of platelets to neutrophils in EDTA anticoagulated blood was described in the 1960s and referred to as *platelet satellitism*.[131–133] This phenomenon was later confirmed in several experiments using whole blood that revealed: platelet agonist-induced aggregates contain both platelets and neutrophils,[134] exposure of whole blood to glass causes deposition of both cell types,[135] and adhesion of neutrophils to nylon fibers increases with increasing platelet concentration.[136] Nash and colleagues observed heterotypic aggregates after mixing heparinized platelet-rich plasma and granulocytes.[137] The response was particularly robust if the platelets were activated. Neutrophil activation also facilitated platelet-leukocyte interactions.

In the late 1980s, a number of investigative groups reported that platelet-leukocyte adhesion was mediated through expression of platelet activation-dependent, granule external membrane protein (PADGEM), currently referred to as P-selectin.[138–140]

The dynamics of platelet-leukocyte interactions in whole blood have been examined.[141] Using RGDS peptides to block platelet aggregation, whole blood was stimulated by thrombin. As expected, this provoked expression of P-selectin (platelet activation). In addition, there was a marked increase in monocyte- and neutrophil-platelet aggregates, as well as an increase in the number of platelets bound per cell. The observed increase in adhesion was blocked using a monoclonal antibody against P-selectin. With thrombin stimulation, monocytes bind more platelets, and at a faster rate, than do neutrophils. With weaker agonists (ADP, epinephrine) less P-selectin is expressed, and whereas platelet-monocyte aggregates are present, neutrophil-platelet conjugates are not.

When whole blood is stimulated with either ADP or epinephrine in the absence of RGDS peptides (thus allowing platelet aggregation), there is a marked decrease in platelet-leukocyte binding and heterotypic platelet aggregates. With time (approximately five minutes), the platelet aggregates spontaneously dissociate and the percentage of monocytes and PMNs with adherent platelets again increase. This subsequent "re-aggregation" is also blocked by the monoclonal antibody G1, supporting P-selectin as the putative receptor.

Genetic polymorphisms in P-selectin ($CD62_p$) and P-selectin glycoprotein ligand-1 (PSGL-1) may reduce platelet-leukocyte aggregate formation (and the response to drug therapy (e.g. Clopidgorel).[142]

Upregulation of VCAM-1, ICAM-1 and E-selectin expression promotes monocyte recruitment to sites of vascular injury. Thrombospondin-1, a protein released from platelets following activation, reduces VCAM- and ICAM-1 expression on endothelial cells, increasing monocyte attachment. The effect is CD47 dependent, supporting an interaction between thrombospondin (platelets), monocytes (CD47 expressing) and injured (or dysfunctional) vascular endothelial cells.[143]

Platelet CD40 and CD40L mediate inflammatory, immunoregulatory and hemostatic functions; each contribute to an evolving and expanded view of platelets as biologic mediators in disease processes, including atherothrombosis, diabetes and inflammatory bowel disease.[144]

Platelet-leukocyte interactions may also be regulated through toll-like receptors (TLR) particularly TLR4.[145]

There is some experimental evidence that the GPIIb/IIIa complex may play a role in the adhesion of activated platelets to leukocytes.[146]

Inflammation and Thrombosis

It was believed previously that thrombosis and inflammation existed at opposite ends of the atherothrombosis spectrum. Growing evidence now links the two processes much more closely. Platelets themselves have been shown to contain several inflammatory mediators and growth factors that play a pivotal role in atherothrombosis; these include CD40 ligand, cyclooxygenase (COX), epithelial neutrophil-activating protein (ENA)-78, interleukin (IL)-1β, macrophage inflammatory protein (MIP)-1α, platelet-derived growth factor (PDGF), platelet factor-4 (PF-4), P-selectin, RANTES (Regulated on Activation, Normal T-Cell Expressed and Secreted) and transforming growth factor-β (TGF-β).

Of the inflammatory molecules described to date, four particularly robust proteins involved with inflammatory processes are the chemokines PF-4, RANTES, MIP-1α and ENA-78.[147] Surface-expressed PF-4 attracts both monocytes and leukocytes and enhances the binding of oxidized LDL (oxLDL) to endothelial and smooth muscle cells.[148] When PF-4 and oxLDL co-localize within foam cells of the atherosclerotic plaque, macrophage esterification of (oxLDL) is intensified.[148] Simultaneously, PF-4 facilitates macrophage differentiation,[147] and participates in the recruitment and activation of monocytes.[149]

RANTES is also a powerful chemoattractant, drawing monocytes and T-lymphocytes to regions of activated platelets. Once secreted, RANTES is deposited by platelets on the endothelial surface, enabling mononuclear cells to be tethered to the disrupted vascular wall.[150] In addition, RANTES directly stimulates genes that regulate inflammatory pathways within monocytes, inducing the synthesis of additional inflammatory mediators, including as IL-8, monocyte chemoattractant protein (MCP)-1, MIP-1α and tumor necrosis factor (TNF)-α.[90,151] Activated platelets not only secrete MIP-1α, a monocyte chemoattractant and macrophage activator,[152] but also induce its synthesis by endothelial cells.[153] This raises the possibility that adhesion of activated platelets to the vascular endothelium may upregulate MIP-1α expression (by endothelial cells), and that MIP-1α, in turn, may fulfill a chemotactic function at the sites of vessel wall injury by activating platelets.

ENA-78 induces β_2 integrin signaling, which greatly increases neutrophil adhesion to the endothelium.[154] It is also synthesized by endothelial cells in response to platelet expression of IL-1β. IL-1β is produced when platelets are activated, and its expression on the platelet membrane triggers production not only of ENA-78, but also of E-selectin and IL-8, each of which facilitate endothelial cell adhesiveness.[147,149]

The role of COX as an important inflammatory mediator in atherothrombosis has been characterized extensively through investigation of aspirin. Platelet activation liberates arachidonic acid from cellular membranes by inducing its phospholipase A_2-mediated hydrolysis. Free arachidonic acid is then metabolized by COX, beginning a biochemical cascade that results in thromboxane A_2 formation (Fig. 5),[155] Two other important molecules that are stored in platelets and provoke inflammation are the transmembrane protein CD40 ligand (CD40L) and P-selectin. CD40L is rapidly cleaved to soluble CD40L following its presentation on the platelet surface.[156] This protein is capable of provoking a number of inflammatory responses by endothelial cells, most notably the production of reactive oxygen species,[157]

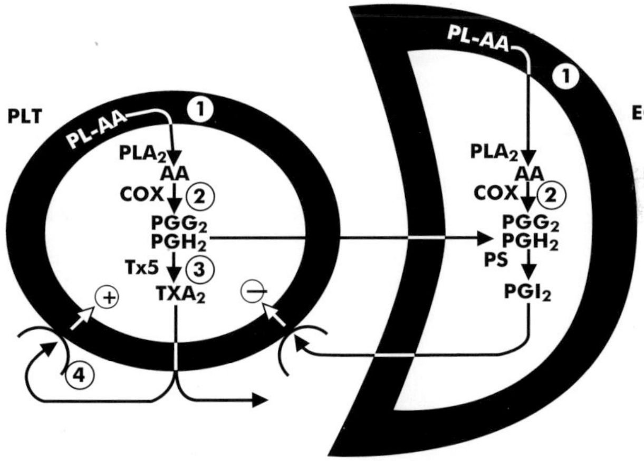

Fig. 5. Interactions between platelets (PLT) and endothelial cells (EC) mediated by arachidonic acid (AA) metabolites. Activators of each cell type induce phospholipase A_2-mediated hydrolysis of free AA from membrane phospholipids (PL) pools. AA is converted by cyclooxygenase (COX) to prostaglandain endoperoxides, PGG_2 and PGH_2. Endoperoxides are metabolized to thromboxane A_2 by prostacyclin synthase in endothelial cells. Thromboxane A_2 binds to platelet receptors to stimulate platelet activation; PGI_2 binds to separate platelet receptors to inhibit platelet activation. With permission from Schafer AI, Antiplatelet therapy, *Am J Med* 1996;**101**:199–209.[155]

chemokines and cytokines (IL-6 and tissue factor),[158] and the expression of adhesion molecules (VCAM-1, ICAM-1 and E-selectin).[159]

Vesicle-stored P-selectin migrates to the platelet's outer membrane during adhesion,[160] where it then engages the P-selectin glycoprotein (PSGL)-1 receptor expressed on leukocytes, enabling leukocytes to roll, adhere (Fig. 6) and eventually transmigrate into the vascular wall.[82] Macrophage accumulation in the vessel wall is also accomplished by P-selectin-mediated amplification of monocyte adhesion to the endothelium.[161] Other proinflammatory functions of P-selectin include upregulation of tissue factor expression on monocytes[162,163] and facilitation of RANTES and PF-4 deposition by platelets.[150]

Two platelet-derived growth factors, PDGF and TGF-β, stimulate the migration and proliferation of vascular smooth muscle cells. PDGF can also be synthesized by macrophages and foam cells, providing potential sources for growth factors found within atherosclerotic lesions.[164]

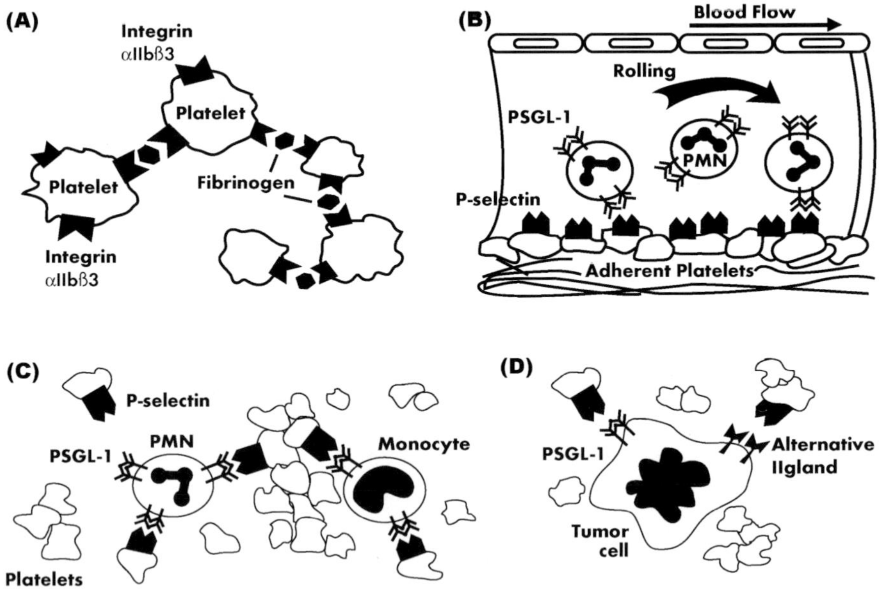

Fig. 6. Rolling of leukocytes (PMN) on adherent, activated platelet mediated via interactions between P-selectin and P-selectin glycoprotein (PSGL-1). With permission from Weyrich AS, Lindemann S, Zimmerman GA, The evolving role of platelets in inflammation, *J Thromb Haemost* 2003;**1**:1897–1905.[147]

Measurable levels of several inflammatory proteins stored within platelets are elevated among patients with coronary artery disease. P-selectin levels correlate with future cardiovascular events in both healthy individuals and patients with suspected myocardial ischemia.[165,166] Similarly, patients with acute coronary syndromes have increased blood levels of both soluble and membrane-bound CD40L.[167]

Platelet RNA and Proteomics

The presence of ribosomes and mRNA molecules within platelets is well established. Traditionally, filtration procedures were used to minimize leukocyte contamination of platelet concentrates. More recent investigations have uncovered hundreds of proteins and gene transcripts within purified platelets with representation of several categories, including surface glycoproteins (integrins), cytoskeletal proteins and functional proteins.[168]

Summary

Platelets are complex circulating cellular elements that contribute both directly and indirectly to hemostasis and atherothrombosis. Their diverse biological effects are governed by increasingly well-characterized anatomic, biochemical, and molecular processes which lay the groundwork for novel diagnostic, prognostic and therapeutic investigations.

References

1. White JG. Platelet ultrastructure. In: Bloom AL, Thomas DP (eds.) *Haemostasis and Thrombosis*, 2nd ed. Churchill Livingston, Edinburgh, 1987, p. 20.
2. George JN. Studies on platelet plasma membranes. IV. Quantitative analysis of platelet membrane glycoproteins by (^{125}1)-diazotized diiodosulfanilic acid labeling and SDS-polycrylamide gel electrophoresis. *J Lab Clin Med* 1978;**92**:430–446.
3. Nurden AT, Caen JP. Membrane glycoproteins and human platelet function. *Br J Haematol* 1978;**38**:155–160.

4. Phillips DR, Agin PP. Platelet membrane defects in Glanzmann's thrombasthenia. Evidence for decreased amounts of two major glycoproteins. *J Clin Invest* 1977;**60**:535–545.
5. Phillips DR, Agin PP. Platelet plasma membrane glycoproteins. Evidence for the presence of none-equivalent disulfide bonds using nonreduced-reduced two-dimensional gel electrophoresis. *J Biol Chem* 1977;**252**:2121–2126.
6. Mann KG, Nesheim ME, Church WR, Hale R, Krishnaswamy S. Surface-dependent relations of the vitamin K-dependent enzyme complexes. *Blood* 1990;**76**:1–16.
7. Tracy PB. Regulation of thrombin generation at cell surfaces. *Semin Thromb Hemost* 1988;**14**:227–233.
8. Zucker-Franklin D. The submembranous fibrils of human blood platelets. *J Cell Biol* 1970;**47**:293–299.
9. White JG. The submembrane filaments of blood platelets. *Am J Pathol* 1969;**56**:267–277.
10. White JG. Effects of colchicine and Vinca alkaloids on human platelets. I. Influence on platelet microtubules and contractile function. *Am J Pathol* 1968;**53**:281–291.
11. Fox JE, Boyles JK, Reynolds CC, Phillips DR. Actin filament content and organization in unstimulated platelets. *J Cell Biol* 1984;**98**:1985–1991.
12. Fox JE. The platelet cytoskeleton. *Thromb Haemost* 1993;**70**:884–893.
13. White JG. Electron microscopic studies of platelet secretion. *Progr Hemost Thromb* 1974;**2**:49–98.
14. White JG. Identification of platelet secretion in the electron microscope. *Ser Haematol* 1973;**6**:429–459.
15. Cutler L, Rodan G, Feinstein MB. Cytochemical localization of adenylate cyclase and of calcium ion, magnesium ion-activated ATPases in the dense tubular system of human blood platelets. *Biochim Biophys Acta* 1978;**542**:357–371.
16. Kaser-Glanzmann R, Jakabove M, George JN, Luscher EF. Further characterization of calcium-accumulating vesicles from human blood platelets. *Biochim Biophys Acta* 1978;**512**:1–12.
17. Weiss HJ. Platelet physiology and abnormalities of platelet function (first of two parts). *N Engl J Med* 1975;**293**:531–541.
18. Plow EF, Ginsberg M. The molecular basis of platelet function. In: Hoffman R, Benz EJ, Shaltil SJ, Furie B, Cohen HJ (eds.) *Hematology. Basic Principles and Practice*. Churchill Livingston, New York, 1991, p. 1165.
19. Roth GJ. Platelets and blood vessels: the adhesion event. *Immunol Today* 1992;**13**:100–105.

20. Fuvel F, Grant ME, Legrand YJ, *et al.* Interaction of blood platelets with a microfibrillar extract from adult bovine aorta: requirement for von Willebrand factor. *Proc Natl Acad Sci USA* 1983;**80**:551–554.
21. Birembaut P, Legrand HY, Bariety J, *et al.* Histochemical and ultrastructural characterization of subendothelial glycoprotein microfibrils interacting with platelets. *J Histochem Cytochem* 1982;**30**:75–80.
22. Roth GJ. Developing relationships: arterial platelet adhesion, glycoprotein Ib, and leucine-rich glycoproteins. *Blood* 1991;**77**:5–19.
23. Turitto VT, Muggli R, Baumgartner HR. Physical factors influencing platelet deposition on subendoethelium: importance of blood shear rate. *Ann NY Acad Sci* 1977;**283**:284–292.
24. Turitto VT, Baumgartner HR. Platelet-surface interactions. In: Colman RW, Hirsh J, Marder VJ, Salzman EW (eds.) *Hemostasis and Thrombosis. Basic Principles and Clinical Practice.* JB Lippincott, Philadelphia, 1987, p. 555.
25. Berridge MJ. Inositol trisphosphate and diacylglycerol: two interacting second messengers. *Annu Rev Biochem* 1987;**56**:159–193.
26. Rink TJ, Sage SO. Calcium signaling in human platelets. *Annu Rev Physiol* 1990;**52**:431–449.
27. Packham MA. Platelet reactions in thrombosis. In: Gottlieb AI, Langilee BL, Federoff S (eds.) *Atherosclerosis. Cellular and Molecular Interactions in the Artery Wall.* Plenum Press, New york, 1991, p. 209.
28. Szasz R, Dale GL. Thrombospondin and fibrinogen bind serotonin-derivatized proteins on COAT-platelets. *Blood* 2005;**100**:2827–2831.
29. Penz S, Reininger AJ, Brandl R, *et al.* Human atheromatous plaques stimulate thrombus formation by activating platelet glycoprotein VI. *FASEB J* 2005;**19**:898–909.
30. Hamilton SF, Miller MW, Thompson CA, Dale GL. Glycoprotein IIb/IIa inhibitors increase COAT-platlet production *in vitro. J Lab Clin Med* 2004;**143**:320–326.
31. Seiler SM, Goldenberg HJ, Michel IM, Hunt JT, Zavoico GB. Multiple pathways of thrombin-induced platelet activation differentiated by desensitization and a thrombin exosite inhibitor. *Biochem Biophys Res Commun* 1991;**181**:636–643.
32. Greco NJ, Jamieson GA. High and moderage affinity pathways for alpha-thrombin-induced platelet activation. *Proc Soc Exp Biol Med* 1991; **198**:792–799.
33. Jamieso GA, Okumura T. Reduced thrombin binding and aggregation in Bernard-Soulier platelets. *J Clin Invest* 1978;**61**:861–864.

34. Wicki AN, Clemetson KJ. Structure and function of platelet membrane glycoproteins Ib and V. Effects of leukocyte elastase and other proteases on platelets response to von Willebrand factor and thrombin. *Eur J Biochem* 1985;**153**:1–11.
35. Cooper HA, Bennett WP, White GC, Wagner H. Hydrolysis of human platelet membrane glycoproteins with a *Serratia marcescens* metalloprotease: effect on response to thrombin and von Willebrand factor. *Proc Natl Acad Sci USA* 1982;**79**:1433–1437.
36. Vu TK, Hung DT, Wheaton VO, Coughlin SR. Molecular cloning of a functional thrombin receptor reveals a novel preoteolytic mechanism of receptor activation. *Cell* 1991;**64**:1057–1068.
37. Vu TK, Wheaton VI, Hung DT, Charo I, Couglin SR. Domains specifying thrombin-receptor interactions. *Nature* 1991;**353**:674–677.
38. Coughlin SR, Vu TKh, Hung DT, Wheaton VI. Characterization of a functional thrombin receptor. Issues and opportunities. *J Clin Invest* 1991;**89**:351–355.
39. Grand RJ, Turnell AS, Grabham PW. Cellular consequences of thrombin-receptor activation. *Biochem J* 1996;**313**:353–368.
40. Coughlin SR. How the protease thrombin talks to cells. *Proc Natl Acad Sci USA* 1999;**96**:11023–11027.
41. Dery O, Corvera CI, Steinhoff M, Bunnett NW. Proteinase-activated receptors: novel mechanisms of signaling by serine proteases. *Am J Physiol* 1998;**274**:C1429–C1452.
42. Nelken NA, Soifer SJ, O'Keefe J, Vu TK, Charo IF, Coughlin SR. Thrombin receptor expression in normal and atherosclerotic human arteries. *J Clin Invest* 1992;**90**:1614–1621.
43. Kaplanski G, Marin V, Fabrigoule M, *et al.* Thrombin-activated human endothelial cells support monocyte adhesion *in vitro* following expression of intercellular adhesion molecule-1 (ICAM-1; CD54) and vascular cell adhesion molecule-1 (VCAM-1; CD106). *Blood* 1998;**92**:1259–1267.
44. Lidington EA, Haskard DO, Mason JC. Induction of decay-accelerating factor by thrombin through a protease-activated receptor 1 and protein kinase C-dependent pathway protects vascular endothelial cells from complement-mediated injury. *Blood* 2000;**96**:2784–2792.
45. Libby P, Sukhova G, Lee RT, Liao JK. Molecular biology of atherosclerosis. *Int J Cardiol* 1997;**62**(Suppl 2):S23–S29.
46. Morris R, Winyard PG, Blake DR, Morris CJ. Thrombin in inflammation and healing: relevance to rheumatoid arthritis. *Ann Rheum Dis* 1994;**53**:72–79.
47. Schini-Kerth VB, Bassus S, Fisslthaler B, Kirchmaier CM, Busse R. Aggregating human platelets stimulate the expression of thrombin receptors

in cultured vascular smooth muscle cells via the release of transforming growth factor-beta1 and platelet-derived growth factor AB. *Circulation* 1997;**96**:3888–3896.

48. Chambers RC, Leoni P, Blanc-Brude OP, Wembridge DE, Laurent GJ. Thrombin is a potent inducer of connective tissue growth factor production via proteolytic activation of protease-activated receptor-1. *J Biol Chem* 2000;**275**:35584–35591.
49. Lova P, Campus F, Lombardi R, *et al.* Contribution of protease-activated receptors 1 and 4 and glycoprotein 1b-1X-V in the Gi-independent activation of platelet Rap1B by thrombin. *J Biol Chem* 2004;**279**:25299–25306.
50. Dubois C, Steiner B, Meyer Reigner SC. Contribution of PAR-1, PAR-4 and GPIbalpha in intracellular signaling leading to the cleavage of the beta3 cytoplasmic domain during thrombin-induced platelet aggregation. *Thromb Haemost* 2004;**91**:733–742.
51. Stenberg PE, Shuman MA, Levine SP, Bainton DF. Redistribution of alpha-granules and their contents in thrombin-stimulated platelets. *J Cell Biol* 1984;**98**:748–760.
52. Ginsberg MH, Taylor L, Painter RG. The mechanism of thrombin-induced platelet factor 4 secretion. *Blood* 1980;**55**:661–668.
53. Holmsen H, Day HJ. The selectivity of the thrombin-induced platelet release reaction: Subcellular localization of released and retained constituents. *J Lab Clin Med* 1970;**75**:840–855.
54. Kenney DM, Chao FC. Microtubule inhibitors alter the secretion of beta-blucoronidase by human blood platelets: involvement of microtubules in release reaction II. *J. Cell Physiol* 1978;**96**:43–52.
55. Holmsen H, Robkin L, Day HJ. Effects of antimycin A and 2-deoxyglucose on secretion in human platelets. Differential inhibition of the secretion of acid hydrolases and adenine nucleotides. *Biochem J* 1979;**182**:413–419.
56. Heldin CH, Westermark B. Platelet-derived growth factor: three isoforms and two receptor types. *Trends Genet* 1989;**5**:108–111.
57. Wenger RH, Wicki AN, Walz A, Kieffer N, Clemetson KJ. Cloning of cDNA coding for connective tissue activating peptide III from a human platelet derived lambda gt II expression library. *Blood* 1989;**73**:1498–1503.
58. Deuel TF, Keim PS, Farmer M, Heinrikson RL, Amino acid sequence of human platelet factor 4. *Proc Natl Acad Sci USA* 1977;**74**:2256–2258.
59. Viskup RW, Tracy PB, Mann KG. The isolation of human platelet factor V. *Blood* 1987;**69**:1188–1195.
60. Rand MD, Kalafatis M, Mann KG. Platelet coagulation factor Va: the major secretory platelet phosphoprotein. *Blood* 1994;**83**:2180–2190.

61. Schwarz HP, Heeb MJ, Wencel-Drake JD, Griffin JH. Identification and quantitation of protein S in human platelets. *Blood* 1985;**66**:1452–1455.
62. Erickson LA, Ginsberg MH, Loskutoff DJ. Detection and partial characterization of an inhibitor of plasminogen activator in human platelets. *J Clin Invest* 1984;**74**:1465–1472.
63. Keenan JP, Solum NO. Quantitative studies on the release of platelet fibrinogen by thrombin. *Br J Haematol* 1972;**23**:461–466.
64. Majack RA, Goodman LV, Dixit VM. Cell surface thrombospondin is functionally essential for vascular smooth muscle cell proliferation. *J Cell Biol* 1988;**106**:415–422.
65. Woods VL Jr, Wolff LE, Keller DM. Resting platelets contain a substantial centrally located pool of glycoprotein IIb-IIIa complex which may be accessible to some but not other extracellular proteins. *J Biol Chem* 1986;**261**:15242–15251.
66. Niija K, Hodson E, Bader R, *et al.* Increased surface expression of the membrane glycoprotein IIb/IIIa complex induced by platelet activation. Relationship to the binding of fibrinogen and platelet aggregation. *Blood* 1987;**70**:475–483.
67. Savage B, Hunger CS, Harker LA, Woods VI Jr, Hanson SR. Thrombin induced increase in surface expression of epitopes on platelet membrane glycoprotein IIb/IIIa complex and GMP-140 is a function of platelet age. *Blood* 1989;**74**:1007–1014.
68. Hellem A. The adhesiveness of human blood platelets *in vitro. Scand J Clin Invest* 1960;**12**:1–117.
69. Gaarder A, Jonsen A, Laland S, Hellem AJ, Owren PA. Adenosine diphosphate in red cells as a factor in the adhesiveness of human blood platelets. *Nature* 1961;**195**:531–532.
70. Burnstock G, Kennedy C. Is there a basis for distinguishing two types of P_2 purinoceptor? *Gen Pharmacol* 1985;**16**:433–440.
71. Fredholm B, Abbracchio MP, Burnstock G, *et al.* Nomenclature and classification of purinoceptors. *Pharmacol Rev* 1994;**46**:143–156.
72. Abbracchio MP, Burnstock G. Purinoceptors: are there three families of P2X and P2Y purinoceptors? *Pharmacol Ther* 1994;**64**:445–475.
73. Nachman RL, Ferris B. Binding of adenosine diphosphate by isolated membranes from human platelets. *J Biol Chem* 1974;**249**:704–710.
74. Cattaneo M, Lecchi A, Randi AM, McGregor JL, Mannucci PM. Identification of a new congenital defect of platelet aggregation characterized by severe impairment of platelet resonse to adenosine diphosphate. *Blood* 1992;**80**:2787–2796.

75. Nurden P, Savi P, Heilmann E, *et al.* An inherited bleeding disorder linked to a defective interaction between ADP and its receptor on platelets. Its influence on glycoprotein IIb-IIIa complex function. *J Clin Invest* 1995;**95**:1612–1622.
76. van de Meijden PE, Feijge MA, Giesen PL, Huijberts M, van Raak LP, Heemskerk JW. Platelet P2Y12 receptors enhance signalling towards procoagulant activity and thrombin generation A study with healthy subjects and patients at thrombotic risk. *Thromb Haemost* 2005:**93**:1128–1136.
77. Altieri DC, Mannucci PM, Capitano AM. Binding of fibrinogen to human monocytes. *J Clin Invest* 1986;**78**:968–976.
78. Feolde E, Vigne P, Breittmayer JP, Frelin C. ATP, a partial agonist of atypical P2Y purinoceptors in rat brain capillary endothelial cells. *Br J Pharmacol* 1995;**115**:1199–1203.
79. Poncz M, Eisman R, Heidenreich R, *et al.* Structure of the platelet membrane glycoprotein IIb: homology to the alpha subunits of the vitronectin and fibronectin membrane receptors. *J Biol Chem* 1987;**262**:8476–8482.
80. Weisel JW, Nagaswami C, Vilaire G, Bennett JS. Examination of the platelet membrane glycoprotein IIb/IIIa complex and its interaction with fibrinogen and other ligands by electron microscopy. *J Biol Chem* 1992;**267**:16637–16643.
81. Hoffman M, A cell-based model of hemostasis. *Thromb Haemost* 2001;**85**:958–965.
82. McEver RP. Adhesive interactions of leukocytes, platelets, and the vessel wall during hemostasis and inflammation. *Thromb Haemost* 2001;**86**:746–756.
83. Monroe DM, Platelets and thrombin generation. *Arterioscler Thromb Vasc Biol* 2002;**22**:1381–1389.
84. Yee DL, Sun CW, Bergeron AL, Dong JF, Bray PF. Aggregometry detects platelet hyperreactivity in healthy individuals. *Blood* 2005;**106**:2723–2729.
85. Packham MA, Guccione MA, Kinlough-Rathbone RL, Mustard JF. Platelet sialic acid and platelet survival after aggregation by ADP. *Blood* 1980;**56**:876–880.
86. Kinlough-Rathbone RL, Packham MA, Guccione MA, Richardson M, Harfenist EJ, Mustard JF. Characteristics of thrombin-degranulated human platelets: development of a method that does not use proteolytic enzymes for deaggregation. *Thromb Haemost* 1991;**65**:403–410.
87. Lindemann S, McIntyre TM, Prescott SM, Zimmerman GA, Weyrich AS. Expanding the functional repertoire of platelets in thrombosis and inflammation: signal-dependent protein synthesis. In: Fitzgerald DJ, Quinn MJ (eds.) *Platelet Function: Assessment, Diagnosis, and Treatment.* The Human Press Inc., Totowa, 2003.

88. Owen WG, Bichler J, Ericson D, Wysokinski W. Gating of thrombin in platelet aggregates by pO_2-linked lowering of extracellular Ca^{2+} concentration. *Biochemistry* 1995;**34**:9277–9281.
89. Lindemann S, Tolley ND, Dixon DA, *et al.* Activated platelets mediate inflammatory signaling by regulated interleukin 1beta synthesis. *J Cell Biol* 2001;**154**:485–490.
90. Weyrich AS, Elstad MR, McEver RP, *et al.* Activated platelets signal chemokine synthesis by human monocytes. *J Clin Invest* 1996;**97**:1525–1534.
91. Galt SW, Lindemann S, Medd D, *et al.* Differential regulation of matrix metalloproteinase-9 by monocytes adherent to collagen and platelets. *Circ Res* 2001;**89**:509–516.
92. Lehr HA, Weyrich AS, Saetzler RK, *et al.* Vitamin C blocks inflammatory platelet-activating factor mimetics created by cigarette smoking. *J Clin Invest* 1997;**99**:2358–2364.
93. Issekutz AC, Ripley M, Jackson JR. Role of neutrophils in the deposition of platelets during acute inflammation. *Lab Invest* 1983;**49**:716–724.
94. Redl H, Hammerschmidt DE, Schlag G. Augmentation by platelets of granulocyte aggregation in response to chemotaxins: studies utilizing an improved cell preparation technique. *Blood* 1983;**61**:125–131.
95. Boogaerts MA, Vercellotti G, Roelant C, Malbrain S, Verwilghen RL, Jacob HS. Platelets augment granulocyte aggregation and cytotoxicity: uncovering of their effects by improved cell separation techniques using Percoll gradients. *Scand J Haematol* 1986;**37**:229–236.
96. De Gaetano G, Evangelista V, Rajtar G, Del Maschio A, Cerletti C. Activated polymorphonuclear leukocytes stimulate platelet function. *Thromb Res Suppl* 1990;**11**:25–32.
97. Oda M, Satouchi K, Yasunaga K, Saito K. Polymorphonuclear leukocyte-platelet interactions: acetylglyceryl ether phosphocholine-induced platelet activation under stimulation with chemotactic peptide. *J Biochem (Tokyo)* 1986;**100**:1117–1123.
98. Coeffier E, Joseph D, Prevost MC, Vargaftig BB. Platelet-leukocyte interaction: activation of rabbit platelets by FMLP-stimulated neutrophils. *Br J Pharmacol* 1987;**92**:393–406.
99. Del Maschio A, Evangelista V, Rajtar G, Chen ZM, Cerletti C, De Gaetano G. Platelet activation by polymorphonuclear leukocytes exposed to chemotactic agents. *Am J Physiol* 1990;**258**:870–879.

100. Fox JE, Lipfert L, Clark EA, Reynolds CC, Austin CD, Brugge JS. On the role of the platelet membrane skeleton in mediating signal transduction. Association of GP IIb-IIIa, pp60c-src, pp62c-yes, and the p21ras GTPase-activating protein with the membrane skeleton. *J Biol Chem* 1993;**268**:25973–29984.
101. Dinerman J, Mehta J, Lawson D, Mehta P. Enhancement of human neutrophil function by platelets: effects of indomethacin. *Thromb Res* 1988;**15**:509–517.
102. Del Maschio A, Corvazier E, Maillet F, Kazatchkine MD, MacLouf J. Platelet dependent induction and amplification of polymorphonuclear leukocyte lysosomal enzyme release. *Br J Haematol* 1989;**72**:329–335.
103. Coeffier F, Delautier D, LeCouedic JP, Chignard M, Denizot Y, Benveniste J. Cooperation between platelets and neutrophils for paf-acether (platelet-activation factor) formation. *J Leukoc Biol* 1990;**47**:234–243.
104. Palmantier R, Borgeat P. Thrombin-activated platelets promote leukotriene B_4 synthesis in polymorphonuclear leukocytes stimulated by physiological agonists. *Br J Pharmacol* 1991;**103**:1909–1916.
105. Spagnuolo PJ, Ellner JJ, Hassid A, Dunn MJ. Thromboxane A2 mediates augmented polymorphonuclear leukocyte adhesiveness. *J Clin Invest* 1980;**66**:406–414.
106. Goldman G, Welbourn R, Klausner JM, Valeri CR, Shepro D, Hechtman HB. Thromboxane mediates diapedesis after ischemia by activation of neutrophil adhesion receptor interactions with basally expressed intercellular adhesion molecule-1. *Circ Res* 1991;**68**:1013–1019.
107. Mugge A, Heistad DD, Densen P, *et al.* Activation of leukocytes with complement C5a is associated with prostanoid-dependent constriction of large arteries in atherosclerotic monkeys *in vivo. Atherosclerosis* 1992;**95**: 211–222.
108. Padgett RC, Heistad DD, Mugge A, Armstrong ML, Piegors DJ, Lopez JA. Vascular responses to activated leukocytes after regression of atherosclerosis. *Circ Res* 1992;**70**:423–429.
109. Mullane KM, Fornabaio D. Thromboxane synthetase inhibitors reduce infarct size by a platelet-dependent, aspirin-sensitive mechanism. *Circ Res* 1988;**62**:668–678.
110. Wargovich TJ, Mehta J, Nichols WW, *et al.* Reduction in myocardial neutrophil accumulation and infarct size following administration of thromboxane inhibitor U-63, 577A. *Am Heart J* 1987;**114**:1078.
111. Huddleston CB, Lupinetti FM, Laws KH, *et al.* The effects of RO-22-4679, a thromboxane synthetase inhibitor on ventricular fibrillation induced by coronary occlusion in conscious dogs. *Circ Res* 1983;**52**:608.

112. Toki Y, Hieda N, Okumura K, *et al.* Myocardial salvage by a novel thromboxane A2 synthetase inhibitor in a canine coronary occlusion-reperfusion model. *Arzneimittelforschung* 1988;**38**:224–227.
113. Grover GJ, Schumacher WA. Effect of the thromboxane receptor antagonist SQ 29,548 on myocardial infarct size in dogs. *J Cardiovasc Pharmacol* 1988;**11**:29–35.
114. Smith EF, 3rd, Griswold DE, Egan JW, Hillegass LM, DiMartino MJ. Reduction of myocardial damage and polymorphonuclear leukocyte accumulation following coronary artery occlusion and reperfusion by the thromboxane receptor antagonist BM 13.505. *J Cardiovasc Pharmacol* 1989;**13**:715–722.
115. Deuel TF, Huang JS. Platelet-derived growth factor. Structure, function, and roles in normal and transformed cells. *J Clin Invest* 1984;**74**:669–676.
116. Deuel TF, Senior RM, Huang JS, Griffin GL. Chemotaxis of monocytes and neutrophils to platelet-derived growth factor. *J Clin Invest* 1982;**69**:1046–1049.
117. Tahara A, Yasuda M, Itagane H, *et al.* Plasma levels of platelet-derived growth factor in normal subjccts and patients with ischemic heart disease. *Am Heart J* 1991;**122**:986–992.
118. Deuel TF, Senior RM, Chang D, Griffin GL, Heinrikson RL, Kaiser ET. Platelet factor 4 is chemotactic for neutrophils and monocytes. *Proc Natl Acad Sci USA* 1981;**78**:4584–4587.
119. Lonky SA, Wohl H. Stimulation of human leukocyte elastase by platelet factor 4. Physiologic, morphologic, and biochemical effects on hamster lungs *in vitro*. *J Clin Invest* 1981;**67**:817–826.
120. Goetzl EJ, Woods JM, Gorman RR. Stimulation of human eosinophil and neutrophil polymorphonuclear leukocyte chemotaxis and random migration by 12-L-hydroxy-5,8,10,14-eicosatetraenoic acid. *J Clin Invest* 1977;**59**:179–183.
121. MacLouf J, de Laclos BF, Borgeat P. Stimulation of leukotriene biosynthesis in human blood leukocytes by platelet-derived 12-hydroperoxy-icosatetraenoic acid. *Proc Natl Acad Sci USA* 1982;**79**:6042–6604.
122. Rhee BG, Hall ER, McIntire LV. Platelet modulation of polymorphonuclear leukocyte shear induced aggregation. *Blood* 1986;**67**:240–246.
123. Boogaerts MA, Yamada O, Jacob HS, Moldow CF. Enhancement of granulocyte-endothelial cell adherence and granulocyte-induced cytotoxicity by platelet release products. *Proc Natl Acad Sci USA* 1982;**79**:7019–7023.
124. Siminiak T, Flores NA, Sheridan DJ. Neutrophil interactions with endothelium and platelets: possible role in the development of cardiovascular injury. *Eur Heart J* 1995;**16**:160–170.

125. Handin RI, Karabin R, Boxer GJ. Enhancement of platelet function by superoxide anion. *J Clin Invest* 1977;**59**:959–965.
126. Levine PH, Weinger RS, Simon J, Scoon KL, Krinsky NI. Leukocyte-platelet interaction. Release of hydrogen peroxide by granulocytes as a modulator of platelet reactions. *J Clin Invest* 1976;**57**:955–963.
127. Weksler BB. Platelets. In: Gallin JI, Godstein IM, Synderman R (eds.) *Inflammation: Basic Principles and Clinical Correlates.* Raven Press, New York, 1988, pp. 543.
128. Mehta P, Mehta J, Lawson D, Krop I, Letts LG. Leukotrienes potentiate the effects of epinephrine and thrombin on human platelet aggregation. *Thromb Res* 1986;**41**:731–738.
129. Zhou W, Javors MA, Olson MS. Platelet-activating factor as an intercellular signal in neutrophil-dependent platelet activation. *J Immunol* 1992;**149**:1763–1769.
130. Nash GB. Adhesion between neutrophils and platelets: a modulator of thrombotic and inflammatory events? *Thromb Res* 1994;**74**(Suppl 1):S3–S11.
131. Field EJ, MacLeod I. Platelet adherence to polymorphs. *Br Med J.* 1963;**2**:388.
132. Kjeldsberg CR, Swanson J. Platelet satellitism. *Blood* 1974;**43**:831–836.
133. Skinnider LF, Musclow CE, Kahn W. Platelet satellitism—an ultrastructural study. *Am J Hematol* 1978;**4**:179–185.
134. Joseph R, Welch KM, D'Andrea G, Riddle JM. Evidence for the presence of red and white cells within "platelet" aggregates formed in whole-blood. *Thromb Res* 1989;**53**:485–491.
135. Banks DC, Mitchell JR. Leucocytes and thrombosis. I. A simple test of leucocyte behaviour. *Thromb Diath Haemorrh* 1973;**30**:36–46.
136. Rasp FL, Clawson CC, Repine JE. Platelets increase neutrophil adherence *in vitro* to nylon fiber. *J Lab Clin Med* 1981;**97**:812–819.
137. Maeda T, Nash GB, Christopher B, Pecsvarady Z, Dormandy JA. Platelet-induced granulocyte aggregation *in vitro*. *Blood Coagul Fibrinolysis* 1991;**2**:699–703.
138. Jungi TW, Spycher MO, Nydegger UE, Barandun S. Platelet-leukocyte interaction: selective binding of thrombin-stimulated platelets to human monocytes, polymorphonuclear leukocytes, and related cell lines. *Blood* 1986;**67**:629–636.
139. Hamburger SA, McEver RP. GMP-140 mediates adhesion of stimulated platelets to neutrophils. *Blood* 1990;**75**:550–554.
140. Larsen E, Celi A, Gilbert GE, *et al.* PADGEM protein: a receptor that mediates the interaction of activated platelets with neutrophils and monocytes. *Cell* 1989;**59**:305–312.

141. Rinder HM, Bonan JL, Rinder CS, Ault KA, Smith BR. Dynamics of leukocyte-platelet adhesion in whole blood. *Blood* 1991;**78**: 1730–1737.
142. Klinkhardt U, Dragutinovic I, Harder S. P-selectin (CD62p) and P-selectin glycoprotein ligand-1 (PSGL-1) polymorphisms: minor phenotypic differences in the formation of platelet-leukocyte aggregates and response to clopidogrel. *Int J Clin Pharmacol Ther* 2005;**43**:255–263.
143. Narizhneva NV, Razorenova OV, Podrez EA, *et al.* Thrombospondin-1 up-regulates expression of cell adhesion molecules and promotes monocyte binding to endothelium. *Faseb J* 2005;**19**:1158–1160.
144. Langer F, Ingersoll SB, Amirkhosravi A, *et al.* The role of CD40 in CD40L- and antibody-mediated platelet activation. *Thromb Haemost* 2005;**93**:1137–1146.
145. Andonegui G, Kerfoot SM, McNagny K, Ebbert KV, Patel KD, Kubes P. Platelets express functional Toll-like receptor-4. *Blood* 2005;**106**:2417–2423.
146. Spangenberg P, Redlich H, Bergmann I, Losche W, Gotzrath M, Kehrel B. The platelet glycoprotein IIb/IIIa complex is involved in the adhesion of activated platelets to leukocytes. *Thromb Haemost* 1993;**70**:514–521.
147. Weyrich AS, Lindemann S, Zimmerman GA. The evolving role of platelets in inflammation. *J Thromb Haemost* 2003;**1**:1897–1905.
148. Nassar T, Sachais BS, Akkawi S, *et al.* Platelet factor 4 enhances the binding of oxidized low-density lipoprotein to vascular wall cells. *J Biol Chem* 2003;**278**:6187–6193.
149. Huo Y, Schober A, Forlow SB, *et al.* Circulating activated platelets exacerbate atherosclerosis in mice deficient in apolipoprotein E. *Nat Med* 2003;**9**:61–67.
150. von Hundelshausen P, Weber KS, Huo Y, *et al.* RANTES deposition by platelets triggers monocyte arrest on inflamed and atherosclerotic endothelium. *Circulation* 2001;**103**:1772–1777.
151. Weyrich AS, McIntyre TM, McEver RP, Prescott SM, Zimmerman GA. Monocyte tethering by P-selectin regulates monocyte chemotactic protein-1 and tumor necrosis factor-alpha secretion. Signal integration and NF-kappa B translocation. *J Clin Invest* 1995;**95**:2297–2303.
152. Adams DH, Lloyd AR. Chemokines: leucocyte recruitment and activation cytokines. *Lancet* 1997;**349**:490–495.
153. Cha JK, Jeong MH, Bae HR, *et al.* Activated platelets induce secretion of interleukin-1beta, monocyte chemotactic protein-1, and macrophage inflammatory protein-1alpha and surface expression of intercellular

adhesion molecule-1 on cultured endothelial cells. *J Korean Med Sci* 2000;**15**:273–278.

154. Imaizumi T, Albertine KH, Jicha DL, McIntyre TM, Prescott SM, Zimmerman GA. Human endothelial cells synthesize ENA-78: relationship to IL-8 and to signaling of PMN adhesion. *Am J Respir Cell Mol Biol* 1997;**17**:181–192.
155. Schafer AI. Antiplatelet therapy. *Am J Med* 1996;**101**:199–209.
156. Hermann A, Rauch BH, Braun M, Schror K, Weber AA. Platelet CD40 ligand (CD40L)—subcellular localization, regulation of expression, and inhibition by clopidogrel. *Platelets* 2001;**12**:74–82.
157. Urbich C, Dernbach E, Aicher A, Zeiher AM, Dimmeler S. CD40 ligand inhibits endothelial cell migration by increasing production of endothelial reactive oxygen species. *Circulation* 2002;**106**:981–986.
158. Henn V, Slupsky JR, Grafe M, *et al.* CD40 ligand on activated platelets triggers an inflammatory reaction of endothelial cells. *Nature* 1998;**391**:591–594.
159. Slupsky JR, Kalbas M, Willuweit A, Henn V, Kroczek RA, Muller-Berghaus G. Activated platelets induce tissue factor expression on human umbilical vein endothelial cells by ligation of CD40. *Thromb Haemost* 1998;**80**:1008–1014.
160. Zimmerman GA. Two by two: the pairings of P-selectin and P-selectin glycoprotein ligand 1. *Proc Natl Acad Sci USA* 2001;**98**:10023–10024.
161. Ramos CL, Huo Y, Jung U, *et al.* Direct demonstration of P-selectin- and VCAM-1-dependent mononuclear cell rolling in early atherosclerotic lesions of apolipoprotein E-deficient mice. *Circ Res* 1999;**84**:1237–1244.
162. Tousoulis D, Davies G, Stefanadis C, Toutouzas P, Ambrose JA. Inflammatory and thrombotic mechanisms in coronary atherosclerosis. *Heart* 2003;**89**:993–997.
163. Wagner DD, Burger PC. Platelets in inflammation and thrombosis. *Arterioscler Thromb Vasc Biol* 2003;**23**:2131–2137.
164. Huo Y, Ley KF. Role of platelets in the development of atherosclerosis. *Trends Cardiovasc Med* 2004;**14**:18–22.
165. Ridker PM, Buring JE, Rifai N. Soluble P-selectin and the risk of future cardiovascular events. *Circulation* 2001;**103**:491–495.
166. Hillis GS, Terregino C, Taggart P, *et al.* Elevated soluble P-selectin levels are associated with an increased risk of early adverse events in patients with presumed myocardial ischemia. *Am Heart J* 2002;**143**:235–241.
167. Aukrust P, Muller F, Ueland T, *et al.* Enhanced levels of soluble and membrane-bound CD40 ligand in patients with unstable angina. Possible

reflection of T lymphocyte and platelet involvement in the pathogenesis of acute coronary syndromes. *Circulation* 1999;**100**:614–620.
168. Bugert P, Dugrillon A, Gunaydin A, Eichler H, Kluter H. Messenger RNA profiling of human platelets by microarray hybridization. *Thromb Haemost* 2003;**90**:738–748.

2 Thromboxane Antagonists

Brian R. Dulin and Steven R. Steinhubl

Introduction

In modern medicine, few disease processes and their pharmaceutical interventions have histories as extensive as do atherothrombosis and antiplatelet drugs. Acetylsalicylic acid (aspirin) has been commercially available for over a century now, and was the first major pharmaceutical agent available in pill form. Although the potential for salicylates to cause a bleeding tendency was initially recognized as early as 1891,[1] almost 100 years of further research were required prior to identifying aspirin's role in inhibiting platelet function through the prevention of thromboxane production and its eventual incorporation as a cornerstone of the treatment and prevention of cardiovascular disease.

Some of the most important cardiovascular trials performed in the last 20 years have studied aspirin, with most finding relative benefits that have been difficult to match by any other pharmaceutical intervention.[2,3] Yet, there remain significant gaps in our understanding of aspirin as an antiplatelet therapy and whether it is the most efficacious way to prevent thromboxane-related platelet activation. This chapter will specifically discuss the role of thromboxane as a platelet agonist, review the clinical data proving the benefit of inhibiting this pathway, and highlight the areas of ongoing research.

Biosynthesis and Function of Thromboxane A_2

Thromboxane A_2 (TXA_2), previously known as rabbit aorta-contracting substance, was first identified in guinea pig lungs during anaphylaxis in the late 1960s.[4] During that same time frame while Hamberg *et al.* were investigating the formation of prostaglandins by sheep seminal vesicles, they discovered the existence of unstable intermediates formed during the conversion of arachidonic acid to prostaglandins. Later studies by this group in the 1970s isolated and identified the intermediate TXA_2 and designated the more stable end-product as thromboxane B_2 (TXB_2), previously known as 8-(1-hydroxy-3-oxopropyl)-9,12L-dihydroxy-5, 10-heptadecadienoic acid (PHD).[5–8] These studies and many others led to the current understanding that arachidonic acid is converted via multiple reactions utilizing oxygen, fatty acid cyclooxygenase (COX) and peroxidase to the intermediates PGG_2 and PGH_2. PGH_2 is then converted via thromboxane synthase to 12-*L*-hydroxy-5,8,10-heptadecatrienoic acid (HHT) plus malondialdehyde (MDA) and TXA_2. TXA_2 is a highly unstable compound that has a 32-second $t_{1/2}$ in aqueous solution before being degraded to the more stable compound, TXB_2. Due to TXA_2 being a well-known inducer of platelet aggregation, vasoconstriction, and more recently a stimulator of smooth muscle cell proliferation and mitogenesis, it has become a major pharmacological target for reduction in cardiovascular disease processes. The prevention of TXA_2 formation via COX inhibition has been the antiplatelet target exploited by aspirin, however in recent history new pharmacologic therapies targeting the thromboxane pathway have arisen. Thromboxane synthase inhibitors and platelet thromboxane receptor antagonist have been explored in hopes of improving upon the efficacy of aspirin with the hope of fewer side effects.

Aspirin

Willow leaves, a natural source of salicylic acid, were listed as an ingredient in drug recipes on clay tablets from the ancient civilizations of Assyria and Babylon over 2000 years ago. Even Hippocrates is credited with using willow bark for relieving the pain associated with childbirth. It was Reverend Edmund Stone, however, who was the first to study and publish his results of the use of willow bark for the treatment of fevers in 1763.[9] Acetylsalicylic acid (aspirin, from the German name **a**cetyl**spir**saure with the addition of the chemical suffix -**in**) was first synthesized in a pure and stable form by Felix Hoffmann, a young chemist at Friedr. Bayer & Company in 1897, and became the first major drug to be sold in tablet form when five grains (approximately equivalent to today's 325 mg dose) was mixed with starch and compressed into a pill. Not long after reports of bleeding problems with salicylates resurfaced. Paul Gibson proposed in 1948 that aspirin might be useful for the prevention of coronary thrombosis, and the following year presented case reports of its success in the treatment of angina.[10,11] L. L. Craven, a primary care physician who had noticed that his tonsillectomy patients who used large doses of Aspergum for pain relief experienced increased bleeding, was the next to study the use of aspirin in the prevention of "coronary occlusion," reporting a 100% success rate among 1,465 asymptomatic males.[12] However, prior to the widespread acceptance of aspirin for the prevention and treatment of thrombotic events, more than anecdotal reports were needed. The first step towards conducting large-scale clinical trials began with the elucidation of aspirin's mechanism of action.

Aspirin's Mechanism of Action

Although the increased bleeding tendencies of aspirin users had been recognized for decades, its inhibitory effect on platelets was not described until the late 1960s. In two studies published simultaneously in the journal *Nature* in 1971, aspirin's ability to inhibit platelet function by preventing prostaglandin synthesis was first described.[13,14] Over the ensuing years it has been shown that aspirin specifically and irreversibly inhibits platelet cyclooxygenase-1 (COX-1) through the acetylation of the amino acid serine at position 529,[15,16] thereby preventing arachidonic acid access to the COX-1 catalytic site through steric hindrance.[17] Because the non-nucleated platelets lack the biosynthetic capabilities necessary to synthesize new protein, the aspirin-induced defect cannot be repaired for the eight- to ten-day life span of the platelet.

During platelet activation the hydrolysis of membrane phospholipids yields arachidonic acid, which is converted to prostaglandin H_2 (PGH_2) by the catalytic activity of the COX enzyme. Prostaglandin H_2 is then converted via thromboxane synthase to thromboxane A_2. Thromboxane A_2 is only one of multiple platelet agonists (Fig. 1), and is synthesized *in vivo* only

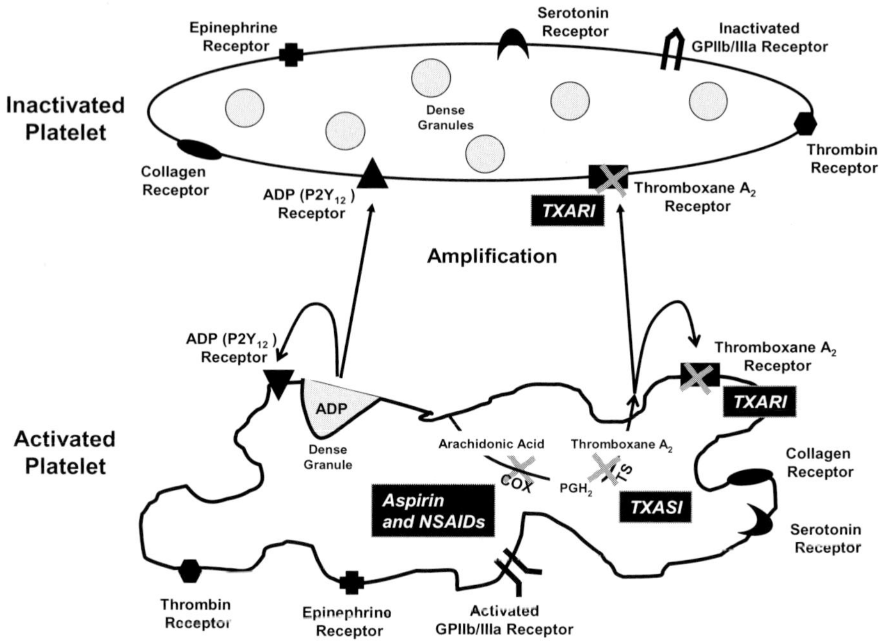

Fig. 1. Multiple sites of platelet activation. Platelet activation leads to synthesis of TXA_2 which is crucial in amplifying the activation process. The sites of action for various classes of thromboxane antagonist antiplatelet agents are shown in black boxes.

by activated platelets. Therefore, by inhibiting thromboxane A_2 synthesis, aspirin does not directly inhibit platelet activation or aggregation, but rather prevents the thromboxane-dependent amplification process that occurs in the setting of a thrombogenic stimulus.

The ability of aspirin to inhibit cyclooxygenase activity, and therefore the production of PGH_2, also accounts for its variety of pharmacologic effects in other tissues. In endothelial cells PGH_2 is the immediate precursor of prostacyclin (PGI_2), which is a vasodilator and inhibitor of platelet aggregation. This counter-balancing effect has raised the concern of a possible prothrombotic effect of aspirin therapy. However, unlike platelets, endothelial cells possess the biosynthetic machinery necessary to produce new enzyme, and therefore recover their ability to synthesize prostacyclin within a few hours. Also, since prostacyclin synthesis by the endothelium is derived by both COX-1 and COX-2,[18] and aspirin is a 170-fold less potent inhibitor of COX-2 than COX-1,[19] adequate *in vivo* prostacyclin production can be maintained despite chronic aspirin therapy. Clinically, no studies have found that higher doses of aspirin therapy are able to initiate a prothrombotic state.

Aspirin in Acute Coronary Syndromes

Although several early, controlled trials of aspirin in patients with a previous myocardial infarction (MI) were able to show trends, at best, toward improved outcomes, no individual trial demonstrated a significant benefit of aspirin over placebo in patients.[20–23] However many of these trials included patients who were relatively remote from their acute coronary syndrome. The first randomized trial to study aspirin in the early treatment of an acute coronary syndrome (within 48 hours of admission for unstable angina) was the Veterans Administration Cooperative Study.[24] In this trial 1266 men with unstable angina were randomized to 324 mg of buffered aspirin daily for 12 weeks or matching placebo. Treatment with aspirin was found to decrease the risk of death or acute MI by 51% (5.0% versus 10.1%, $p = 0.0005$). Three subsequent placebo-controlled trials reinforced the findings of this initial study with a consistent 50% or greater risk reduction in the combined endpoint of death or MI through the early initiation of aspirin therapy.[25–27]

The Second International Study of Infarct Survival (ISIS-2) unequivocally established the beneficial role of aspirin in patients experiencing an ST-elevation MI.[2] In this trial 17,187 patients, admitted within 24 hours after the onset of a suspected acute MI, were randomized to streptokinase (1.5 MU) alone, aspirin (162.5 mg daily for 30 days) alone, both, or neither. Patients receiving aspirin alone experienced a significant 23% relative reduction in vascular mortality during the five weeks following admission compared with those receiving placebo tablets (9.4% versus 11.8%, $p < 0.00001$), with randomization to streptokinase being associated with a similar 25% reduction in 5-week mortality (9.2% for streptokinase versus 12.0% for placebo infusion, $p < 0.00001$). The greatest benefit however was found in patients treated with the combination of aspirin plus streptokinase. This cohort experienced a 42% reduction in vascular mortality compared to placebo allocated patients (8.0% versus 13.2%, $p < 0.00001$), and was significantly better than either active therapy alone.

Aspirin in Secondary Prevention

Despite the compelling evidence from a number of trials supporting the use of aspirin in the early treatment of patients suffering an acute coronary syndrome, results from placebo-controlled trials looking at only the long-term benefit of aspirin in patients who have experienced a remote MI have been less persuasive. The largest of these trials was the Aspirin Myocardial Infarction Study (AMIS), which compared the effects of 1 g of aspirin daily versus placebo in 4524 patients who had experienced at least one previous MI.[21] No significant difference in the primary endpoint of three-year mortality was found and in fact there was a trend in favor of placebo. Several other trials, evaluating aspirin alone, or aspirin plus persantine versus placebo found trends toward mortality benefit with long-term antiplatelet therapy, but no statistically significant benefit.[28–30] However, when the Antiplatelet Trialists analyzed the results of all 11 placebo-controlled post-MI trials, which included just under 20,000 patients, they found a significant benefit of aspirin in terms of recurrent non-fatal MI (4.7% versus 6.5%, $p < 0.00001$) and vascular death (8.1% versus 9.4%, $p < 0.005$).[31] Based on these results, and the evidence for benefit in the primary prevention population, chronic antiplatelet therapy is recommended in virtually all patients who have experienced a thrombotic coronary event. However, the degree of benefit in relation to any potential adverse effects of long-term aspirin in this population must be considered.

Aspirin in Primary Prevention

To date, seven placebo-controlled, randomized trials designed to evaluate the role of long-term aspirin therapy in the primary prevention of death and MI have been reported (Table 1). These trials have included over 96,000 patients at variable risk for future cardiac events and have studied aspirin doses ranging from 75 to 500 mg daily. In the first two studies, the US Physicians' Health Study and the British Doctors' Trial,[32,33] a combined 27,210

Table 1. Randomized, controlled trials of aspirin for primary prevention of death, myocardial infarction and stroke.

Trial	Patients	Aspirin dose	Duration of follow-up	Total mortality, aspirin RR	Non-fatal MI, aspirin RR	Stroke, aspirin RR
Physicians Health Study[114]	22,071 healthy male physicians	325 mg every other day	5 years	0.96	0.59*	1.22
British Doctors' Trial[115]	5139 healthy male physicians	500 mg daily	6 years	0.89	0.97	1.15
Swedish Angina Pectoris Aspirin Trial[39]	2035 males and females with chronic stable angina	75 mg daily	4.2 years	0.78	0.61*	0.75
Thrombosis Prevention Trial[116]	5085 "high-risk" males	75 mg (controlled release preparation) daily	6.4 years	1.06	0.68*	0.98
Hypertension Optimal Treatment Study[117]	18,790 males and females with hypertension	75 mg daily	3.8 years	0.93	0.64*,†	0.98
Primary Prevention Project[118]	4495 male and female with one or more risk factors	100 mg daily	3.6 years	0.81	0.69	0.67
Women's Health Study[38]	39,876 female healthy health care professionals	100 mg every other day	10 years	0.95	1.02	0.83

Risk Ratio (RR) is for aspirin versus placebo.

* Indicates a statistically significant difference between aspirin- and placebo-treated patients.

† Includes all clinically identified myocardial infarctions.

male physicians made up the study group. The results of these trials, involving relatively low-risk, health-conscious individuals, were mixed. Whereas the British study found no significant benefit of aspirin, the larger US trial found that aspirin conferred a significant 44% decrease in the risk of a first MI, although no overall benefit in reducing cardiovascular mortality was found. An increased risk of hemorrhagic stroke was a worrisome finding in both studies. In subsequent primary prevention studies, all utilizing lower doses of aspirin, individuals randomized to active therapy actually experienced a lower incidence of stroke.[34–37] Although there was a trend in most studies towards decreased mortality with aspirin, the results were not statistically significant.

Further information specifically addressing the benefits and risks of aspirin as primary prevention therapy in women was recently addressed in the Women's Health Study.[38] This trial involving 39,876 US female health care professionals 45 years of age or older taking a low dose regimen (100 mg every other day) of aspirin demonstrated that aspirin had no significant effect on the risk of non-fatal MI ($RR = 1.02$; $p = 0.83$) or death ($RR = 0.95$; $p = 0.68$). The study did note a 17% reduction in the risk of stroke versus placebo ($RR = 0.83$; $p = 0.04$). However, upon further subgroup analysis women 65 years of age or older obtained the greatest benefit from aspirin therapy in the reduction of MI, ischemic stroke, and major cardiovascular events. The most noted side effect in the aspirin versus placebo study population was GI bleeding ($RR = 1.4$; $p = 0.02$).

Clearly the level of benefit with aspirin for primary prevention is dependent upon the level of risk for the patient being treated to experience a serious thrombotic event. In the US Physicians' Study, the event rate in the placebo arm was only 0.7% per year. Although a protective effect of aspirin was seen in this study, 250 individuals of equally low risk would need to be treated with aspirin for five years in order to prevent one major vascular event. However, in a cohort of patients with chronic stable angina, such as those studied in the Swedish Angina Pectoris Aspirin Trial (SAPAT)[39] in which the annual event rate was over five times that of patients in the US Physicians' Study, only 91 patients would need to be treated for just one year to prevent a major vascular event. The degree of benefit that an individual may derive from chronic aspirin therapy must also be weighed against the risk of an adverse effect of the therapy, in particular gastrointestinal bleeding.

Aspirin in Percutaneous Coronary Interventions

Antiplatelet therapy has been a critical component of adjunctive medical therapy during percutaneous coronary intervention (PCI) since the inception of this technique over 20 years ago.[40] In these initial patients the use of aspirin and its three-day duration of treatment were empiric. Subsequent placebo-controlled studies established the importance of early aspirin use in PCIs, with the addition of aspirin to full anticoagulation with heparin compared to heparin alone decreasing the risk of Q-wave MI by over 75%.[41,42] Although initial hopes that treatment with aspirin following PCI might impact upon neointimal hyperplasia were not realized, chronic antiplatelet therapy became standard of therapy following PCI due to its proven benefit in secondary prevention and one randomized trial highlighting a benefit of continuing aspirin beyond the acute phase of a coronary intervention.[43]

Aspirin Pharmacodynamics and Dosing

Inhibition of thromboxane-dependent platelet aggregation occurs rapidly after the ingestion of aspirin. Although peak levels of acetylsalicylic acid are achieved within 15 to 20 minutes,[44] platelet function is affected within minutes due to portal circulation exposure of platelets.[45] Chewing an aspirin or using an aspirin solution minimizes the time to maximal inhibition of thromboxane synthesis to approximately 20 minutes, whereas swallowing an enteric-coated aspirin whole delays maximal antiplatelet effects by two to four hours.[44,46] A loading dose of 300 mg is needed to rapidly inhibit thromboxane synthesis by more than 99%.[47] Although the plasma half-life of aspirin is only 20 minutes, since platelets cannot synthesize new cyclooxygenase the effect of aspirin remains for the life of the platelet (approximately ten days). Therefore once aspirin therapy is stopped, ten days are required for complete renewal of platelets, but hemostasis may return to normal with as little as 20% of platelets having normal COX activity.[48] Once platelet thromboxane biosynthesis has been blocked, relatively low doses of chronic aspirin are required to maintain chronic suppression of thromboxane-dependent platelet aggregation. Studies in healthy volunteers have found that a daily maintenance dose of 30 to 40 mg is sufficient to inhibit platelet thromboxane A_2 production and platelet aggregation.[47,49,50]

Dosing recommendations based on the above pharmacodynamic data are restricted by the small number of individuals studied and the implication that there is a uniform response by all individuals to a given dose of aspirin, which is likely, inaccurate.

Clinical trials of aspirin have studied doses ranging from 30 to 1500 mg daily, with no indication of a dose effect. A meta-analysis reviewing aspirin dosing in 11 randomized, placebo-controlled trials involving almost 10,000 patients concluded that all doses from 50 to 1500 mg daily produced the same reduction in stroke risk (15%) in patients with a history of cerebrovascular disease.[51] In another meta-analysis involving over 30,000 patients enrolled in primary prevention trials, high-dose aspirin (600 to 1500 mg daily) was found to be no more efficacious than low-dose (500 mg or less), with the trend favoring low dose.[52] One randomized trial of aspirin dosing in patients undergoing carotid endarterectomy concluded that patients taking 325 mg or less of aspirin had fewer adverse events within three months than did the patients taking 650–1300 mg of aspirin daily.[53]

A synthesis of the available pharmacodynamic and clinical data would suggest that in order to achieve aspirin's maximal antiplatelet effects, at least 300 mg should be chewed or drank as a solution. For the chronic maintenance of aspirin's antiplatelet protection, while minimizing side effects, 40 mg daily seems optimal.

Aspirin Resistance

The phrase "Aspirin Resistance" is a generic term that has been applied to a multitude of clinical and laboratory scenarios. It is generally defined as a lack of response to therapy as determined by the failure to produce expected *ex vivo* results (i.e. specific, frequently arbitrary levels of platelet inhibition). Occasionally, but not consistently, such a measurement has been correlated with the occurrence of thrombotic events. One group performed a study of 180 stroke patients, measuring platelet reactivity 12 hours after the administration of 500 mg of aspirin and found 33% to be "non-responsive" to aspirin.[54] After two years of follow-up, these patients were found to have a ten-fold increased risk of recurrent stroke, MI or death compared to patients identified as aspirin-sensitive at baseline. More recently, investigators evaluated aspirin responsiveness by measuring urinary 11-dehydro-TXB2 (11-dTXB2) levels in a case-control analysis including 488 patients from the Heart Outcomes Prevention Evaluation (HOPE) trial who experienced an MI, stroke, or death. The study found that increasing quartiles of urinary 11-dTXB2 levels were associated with increasing risk of thrombotic events, with patients in the highest quartile having a 1.8-fold increase compared to age- and gender-matched controls.[55] A prospective, blinded analysis also demonstrated the possibility of aspirin resistance by evaluating the aspirin responsiveness, via platelet aggregation and the Platelet Function Analyzer (PFA)-100, of 326 patients with stable cardiovascular disease taking 325 mg of aspirin per day. The study classified 17 (5.2%) of the patients as aspirin resistant and 309 (94.8%) as either sensitive or partially responsive by aggregometry.[56] After a mean of 1.9 years of follow-up, the group of patients classified as aspirin resistant was found to have a significant increase in the risk of death, MI, or stroke. Interestingly, aspirin responsiveness as determined by the PFA-100 had no association with clinical outcomes. A more recent report using the point-of-care Ultegra VerifyNow showed that of the 151 patients scheduled for non-urgent PCI, those patients classified as aspirin resistant had a 2.9-fold increased incidence of creatine kinase (CK)-MB elevation after PCI.[57] Based on the above, all we can estimate is that the prevalence of aspirin resistance ranges from as low as 5% and up to 75% with relatively similar patient populations.[55,56]

A major limitation of virtually all studies reporting an association between measured aspirin responsiveness and clinical outcomes is that they have not truly measured aspirin responsiveness, but rather the platelet function of patients already taking aspirin. As there is marked variability in platelet function among individuals even before antiplatelet therapy, which correlates with the risk of future thrombotic events, it is unclear what effect — that of aspirin on platelet function, baseline platelet function, or a combination of both — that is most predictive of future risk.

There is much that still remains to be learned about the clinical importance and therapeutic options available to patients determined to have an "inadequate" response to aspirin. Currently, there is no proven method to measure clinically meaningful variability in response to aspirin, nor are there alternative therapies proven to improve outcomes. However, it is clear that there is substantial inter-individual variability in the *ex vivo* response to a set dose of aspirin and that ongoing studies will eventually help clarify the issues that have to date made the concept of aspirin resistance primarily an academic curiosity.

Aspirin and NSAIDs

The ability of concomitant non-steroidal anti-inflammatory drugs (NSAIDs) to prevent the antiplatelet effects of aspirin is one mechanism of "aspirin resistance" that has been well described. In the initial landmark study, Catella-Lawson and colleagues demonstrated that when the non-selective COX inhibitor ibuprofen was taken prior to aspirin, aspirin's ability to inhibit serum thromboxane B_2 formation and platelet aggregation was prevented.[58] Acetaminophen, diclofenac and rofecoxib did not share this effect. The postulated mechanism behind this interaction is that ibuprofen, when taken prior to aspirin, blocks the platelet COX-1 catalytic site, and therefore prevents aspirin from accessing the enzyme and irreversibly acetylating the serine residue at position 529. Normally, when aspirin is able to acetylate platelet COX-1, the enzyme is inhibited for the life of the platelet. Ibuprofen on the other hand, a reversible, competitive COX inhibitor is only able to inhibit COX-1 for several hours, and by six hours thromboxane production returns and platelet aggregation begins to approach normal levels. Since aspirin has a very short plasma half-life of only 15 to 20 minutes,[59,60] if acetylation of COX-1 is prevented by ibuprofen during this time, acetylation cannot occur and platelet function will return to normal as soon as $\sim$20% of platelet COX-1 activity returns.[61] A recent study of naproxen confirmed that it also prevents the acetylation of platelet COX-1 by aspirin.[62] Adequately powered clinical trials are still needed to establish the cardiovascular risks and benefits of concomitant aspirin and NSAID therapy.

Adverse Effects of Aspirin

The most frequent side effect associated with aspirin is gastrointestinal (GI) intolerance. Aspirin causes gastric mucosal damage due to a direct toxic effect as well as through the inhibition of cytoprotective prostaglandins. In a meta-analysis of 24 randomized, placebo-controlled trials with almost 66,000 participants the incidence of GI hemorrhage was 2.47% for aspirin-treated patients compared with 1.42% for those taking placebo (odds ratio 1.68, 95% CI 1.51 to 1.88).[63] The risk of GI bleeding with aspirin appears to be dose related, with no common dose, even 75 mg a day, found to be free of risk.[64] Enteric-coating and buffered preparations are better tolerated and have fewer side effects but do not appear to decrease the risk of GI bleeding.[65,66]

Much less frequent, but even more concerning is the risk of hemorrhagic stroke associated with aspirin therapy. Several early trials suggested an increased risk of hemorrhagic stroke with long-term aspirin treatment, but none had the statistical power to provide definitive results. A meta-analysis of 16 trials with 55,462 patients found an absolute increase in the risk of hemorrhagic stroke of 12 events for every 10,000 individuals treated with aspirin (95% CI, 5–20; $p < 0.001$).[67] Importantly, no patient or clinical characteristics were found to be predictive of the risk for hemorrhagic stroke, and although trials were analyzed that used doses ranging from 75 to 1500 mg daily, no clear dose relationship was found.

NO-Aspirin

The past two to three decades has yielded great strides into our knowledge about nitric oxide (NO) as a very complicated biological molecule, endogenously produced in the cardiovascular system by endothelial cells, SMCs, macrophages, neutrophils, and platelets.[68] Numerous studies have demonstrated a wide range of roles played by NO and have found that NO is dependent upon both cGMP-independent (inhibition of cell proliferation, apoptosis, cytokine synthesis inhibition) and cGMP-dependent mechanisms (platelet aggregation inhibition, vasodilation, leukocyte adhesion to endothelium inhibition, increase vascular permeability, antioxidant effects) to exert its biological effects.[69–83] NO has also been found to exert a multitude of effects on the cardiovascular system and in combination with aspirin leads to inhibition of platelet activation and aggregation during clot formation. NO-aspirin exerts its effects both with the aspirin and

NO components of the drug. Aspirin retains its parent drug properties after enzymatic digestion from the ester-linked NO-moiety. Animal models have shown that NO-aspirin has a more pronounced antithrombotic effect than aspirin alone and has been shown to exert cardiovascular protective effects both peripherally and centrally via mechanisms beyond solely inhibiting platelet activation and aggregation.[84–88] In addition to the antiplatelet effects exerted by NO-aspirin, the combined moieties have been shown to provide cardioprotective effects against arrhythmias and reduce infarct size in various animal models.[89,90] Further trials are warranted to investigate the potential additive benefits of the addition of an NO moiety to conventional aspirin therapy.

Thromboxane Synthase Antagonist

Thromboxane synthase is an enzyme belonging to the P450 superfamily associated with endoplasmic reticulum. Thromboxane synthase was viewed as a potentially better therapeutic target than standard cyclooxygenase inhibitors due to further downstream inhibition in the arachidonic acid pathway. Theoretically, accumulation of PGH_2 secondary to thromboxane synthase inhibition might also lead to increased synthesis of the antiaggregatory/vasodilator prostacyclin PGI_2. Based on this a multitude of thromboxane synthase antagonists (TXASIs) have been developed, including ozagrel (OKY-046), pirmagrel (CGS-13080), dazoxiben (UK-37248), (OKY-1581), isbogrel (CV-4151), furegrelate (U-63557A), dazmagrel, CS-518, and camonagrel (Table 2). Numerous clinical trials of TXASI have been performed but have to date yielded relatively disappointing results. One possible reason for this is that several clinical studies have found incomplete inhibition of TXA_2 production by TXASIs.[91] Other potential explanations for these disappointing results include accumulation of PGH_2, which is more stable than TXA_2 and thought to compete with TXA_2 for receptor sites and possess similar pharmacological properties.[8,92–96] Later studies also revealed that TXASIs were not as selective as originally imagined due to their ability to inhibit other cytochrome P450 enzymes and nitric oxide synthase.

Table 2. Selection of thromboxane synthase antagonists, thromboxane receptor antagonists and dual thromboxane synthase and receptor antagonists.

	Drug	Patients	Clinical Evaluation	Results
Thromboxane synthase antagonist	Dozoxiben[119–122]	Healthy volunteers	Platelet aggregation	Weak or no effect
	Primagrel[123]	Healthy volunteers	Platelet aggregation	No effect
	Furegrelate[124]	Healthy volunteers	Platelet aggregation	Variable inhibition
	Dozoxiben[125–129]	Stable angina	Hemodynamic benefit	No benefit to moderate improvement
	Pirmagrel[130]	Peripheral vascular disease	TXA_2 synthesis inhibition	Incomplete inhibition
Thromboxane receptor antagonist	Linotroban[105]	Healthy volunteers	Platelet aggregation	Variable inhibition
	GR 32191B[131]	Human radial artery segments	Vasoconstriction	Reduced vasoconstriction
	Z 335[132]	Healthy volunteers	Platelet aggregation	Variable inhibition
	S 18886[102]	CAD	Flow-mediated vasodilation	Improved
	Ramatroban[104]	Hypercholesterolemic rabbits	Neointimal formation after balloon injury	Downregulated
Dual thromboxane antagonist	Picotamide[106]	Type 2 diabetics with peripheral arterial disease	Two-year mortality	Reduced
	KDI-792[107]	Type 2 diabetics	Lower limb blood flow	Increased
	Terbogrel[108]	Healthy volunteers	Platelet aggregation	Variable inhibition
	Ridogrel[111]	AMI (RAPT trial)	Reinfarction, recurrent angina, ischemic stroke	Decreased by post-hoc analysis
	BM-573[133]	Pig animal model	Coronary thrombosis induced MI	Protective

Thromboxane Receptor Antagonist

Thromboxane receptors (TP) (sometimes referred to as TXA_2/PGH_2 receptors) have been described as playing a variety of roles in biological functions such as hemostasis, thrombosis, hypertension, acute MI, cardiovascular disease, asthma, inflammatory lung disease, chronic inflammatory diseases, lupus nephritis, regulation of acquired immunity, and many more. The seven-transmembrane G-protein-coupled receptor for TXA_2 has two known isoforms designated as TPα and TPβ. The two isoforms exist in various ratios throughout tissue and various cell lines in the body. Messenger RNA for both TPα and TPβ have been isolated in platelets, however, TPα has been shown to be the predominant form.[97,98] Although most biological functions and responses are regulated via multiple pathways, some individual signaling pathways have been suggested to cause specific responses in platelets. In order to inhibit the multitude of TP-mediated G-protein signaling cascades at a common pathway, thromboxane receptor antagonists (TXARIs) were developed. TXARIs are generally classified into two groups based on their structure: prostanoid and non-prostanoid. Some notable TXARIs include: ifetroban, vapiprost, SQ 29548, daltroban, linotroban (HN-11 500), Z 335, S 18886, PTA_2, BM 13177, sulotroban, GR 32191, domitroban, LCB 2853, seratrodast (AA 2414), 13-APA, ONO-3708, SQ 28668, ramatroban (Bay U3405), EP 045, BMS 180291, and S 145 (Table 2). Early animal studies involving TXARIs demonstrated positive antithrombotic and cardioprotective effects.[99–101] Unfortunately, many of the TXARIs did poorly in phase II–III clinical trials and were abandoned for further development. For example, the M-HEART II trial compared sulotroban versus placebo and aspirin in 752 patients for six months following a balloon angioplasty. Aspirin was found to be significantly better than sulotroban and placebo at preventing the combined endpoint of death, MI or clinical restenosis. However, in more recent animal and some human studies newer TXARIs have been shown to inhibit platelet activation/aggregation, inhibit TXA_2-mediated vasoconstriction, improve flow-mediated vasodilation, act as an anti-asthmatic, and downregulate neointimal formation after balloon injury.[102–105]

Dual Thromboxane Synthase/Receptor Antagonist (Modulators)

The unexpected clinical results of the TXASIs and TXARIs have led to the exploration of combined thromboxane synthase/platelet thromboxane receptor antagonist (modulators) pharmaceuticals. The combined thromboxane modulators hope to exploit the positive antiaggregatory and vasodilatory properties of TXASIs and maintain the desired inhibition of TXA_2 and PGH_2 at the receptor level utilizing TXARIs. Based on this principle a number of thromboxane modulators have been developed: ridogrel, picotamide, BM-531, BM-567, samixogrel, BM-573, terbogrel, BM-613, KDI-792, BM-591, and MED 27 (Table 2). Many of these combinatorial pharmaceuticals have undergone animal and human studies. Picotamide was recently evaluated against aspirin in the Drug Evaluation in Atherosclerotic Vascular Disease in Diabetics (DAVID) study, involving type 2 diabetics with peripheral arterial disease and was found to reduce two-year mortality in that patient group.[106] The thromboxance modulator, KDI-792, has been shown to increase lower limb blood flow in type 2 diabetics.[107] Terbogrel, a derivative of samixogrel, is currently under evaluation as an antithrombotic/antiplatelet agent.[108] However, one study evaluating the use of terbogrel in patients with primary pulmonary hypertension was stopped due to the side effect of leg pain being experienced primarily by patients in the terbogrel test group.[109,110] Ridogrel was one of the earliest combined thromboxane modulators studied but did not yield the desired antithrombotic/antiplatelet results. Ridogrel was compared to aspirin as an adjunct to thrombolysis with streptokinase in patients with acute MI in the the Ridogrel Versus Aspirin Patency Trial (RAPT).[111] The study demonstrated similar proportions of patients with a patent infarct-related vessel, clinical markers of reperfusion at two hours post-procedure, and major clinical events during hospitalization between the two study groups. However, post-hoc analysis of the RAPT trial demonstrated a decreased incidence of new ischemic events (defined as reinfarction, recurrent angina, ischemic stroke) in the ridogrel group. Recently, ridogrel has also been evaluated for the possible treatment of ulcerative colitis and inflammatory bowel disease.[112,113] Based on the above results and the possibility of improved efficacy by exploiting the positive effects of both TXASIs and TXARIs, the combined thromboxane modulators may represent a new era of antithrombotic agents. However, further clinical studies are needed to fully investigate their potential clinical applications and side effects.

Conclusion

Chronic oral antiplatelet therapy, in particular the inhibition of platelet thromboxane production by aspirin, is the principal line of defense against thrombotic arterial events. These events are not only the primary cause of death in industrialized nations today, but their incidence continues to increase world wide. Despite our long history of aspirin use, and the global implications of cardiovascular disease, we have yet to discover how to optimally and predictably inhibit the adverse affects of thromboxane on platelets. As our understanding of the diverse role thromboxane plays in influencing platelet function and vascular hemostasis continues to increase, so will our ability to prevent atherothrombotic complications. Currently, our treatment options for the prevention of thromboxane-induced platelet activation are limited, yet as demonstrated in this chapter new agents continue to be developed and current agents will be perfected. Hopefully such progress will translate into even greater benefits than already realized with these agents, and even more lives saved.

References

1. Binz C. *Vorlesungen Ueber Pharmakologie*, 2nd ed. Berlin, 1891.
2. ISIS-2 (Second International Study of Infarct Survival) Collaborative Group. Randomized trial of intravenous streptokinase, oral aspirin, both, or neither among 17,187 cases of suspected acute myocardial infarction; ISIS-2. *Lancet* 1988;**2**:349–360.
3. Wallentin LC, the RISC Group. Aspirin (75 mg/day) after an episode of unstable coronary artery disease: long-term effects on the risk of myocardial infarction, occurrence of severe angina and the need for revascularization. *J Am Coll Cardiol* 1991;**18**:1587–1593.
4. Piper PJ, Vane JR. Release of additional factors in anaphylaxis and its antagonism by anti-inflammatory drugs. *Nature* 1969;**223**(201):29–35.

5. Hamberg M, Samuelsson B. Detection and isolation of an endoperoxide intermediate in prostaglandin biosynthesis. *Proc Natl Acad Sci USA* 1973;**70**(3):899–903.
6. Hamberg M, Samuelsson B. Prostaglandin endoperoxides. Novel transformations of arachidonic acid in human platelets. *Proc Natl Acad Sci USA* 1974;**71**(9):3400–3404.
7. Hamberg M, Svensson J, Samuelsson B. Thromboxanes: a new group of biologically active compounds derived from prostaglandin endoperoxides. *Proc Natl Acad Sci USA* 1975;**72**(8):2994–2998.
8. Hamberg M, *et al.* Isolation and structure of two prostaglandin endoperoxides that cause platelet aggregation. *Proc Natl Acad Sci USA* 1974;**71**(2): 345–349.
9. Stone E. An account of the success of the bark of the willow in the cure of agues. *Philos Trans R Soc Lond [Biol]* 1763;**53**:195–200.
10. Gibson P. Salicylic acid for coronary thrombosis? *Lancet* 1948;**1**:965.
11. Gibson PC. Aspirin in the treatment of vascular diseases. *Lancet* 1949; **2**:1172–1174.
12. Craven LL. Experiences with aspirin (acetylsalicylic acid) in the non-specific prophylaxis of coronary thrombosis. *Miss Valley Med J* 1953;**75**:38–44.
13. Vane JR. Inhibition of prostaglandin synthesis as a mechanism of action for aspirin-like drugs. *Nature New Biol* 1971;**231**:231–235.
14. Smith JB, Willis AL. Aspirin selectively inhibits prostaglandin production in human platelets. *Nature New Biol* 1971;**231**:235–237.
15. Funk C, *et al.* Human platelet/erythroleulemia cell prostaglandin G/H synthase: cDNA cloning, expression and gene chromosomal assignment. *FASEB J* 1991;**5**:2304–2312.
16. Roth G, Stanford N, Majerus P. Acetylation of prostaglandin synthase by aspirin. *Proc Natl Acad Sci USA* 1975;**72**:3073–3076.
17. Loll P, Picot D, Garavito R. The structural basis for aspirin activity inferred from the crystal structure of inactivated prostaglandin H_2 synthase. *Nature (Struct Biol)* 1995;**2**:637–643.
18. McAdam B, *et al.* Systemic biosynthesis of prostacyclin by cyclooxygenase (COX)-2; the human pharmacology of a selective inhibitor of COX-2. *Proc Natl Acad Sci USA* 1999;**96**:272–277.
19. Vane JR, Bakhle YS, Botting RM. Cyclooxygenases 1 and 2. *Ann Rev Pharmacol Toxicol* 1998;**38**:97–120.
20. Breddin K, *et al.* Secondary prevention of myocardial infarction. A comparison of acetylsalicylic acid, placebo and phenprocoumon. *Haemostasis* 1980;**9**:325–344.

21. Aspirin Myocardial Infarction Study Research Group. A randomized, controlled trial of aspirin in persons recovered from myocardial infarction. *JAMA* 1980;**243**:661–669.
22. Elwood P, Sweetnam P. Aspirin and secondary mortality after myocardial infarction. *Lancet* 1979;**2**:1313–1315.
23. Elwood P, *et al.* A randomized controlled trial of acetyl salicylic acid in the secondary prevention of mortality from myocardial infarction. *BMJ* 1974;**1**(905):436–440.
24. Lewis Jr, HD, *et al.* Protective effects of aspirin against acute myocardial infarction and death in men with unstable angina: results of a Veterans Administration Cooperative Study. *N Engl J Med* 1983;**309**:396–403.
25. Cairns JA, *et al.* Aspirin, sulfinpyrazone, or both in unstable angina. *N Engl J Med* 1985;**313**:1369–1375.
26. The RISC Group. Risk of myocardial infarction and death during treatment with low dose aspirin and intravenous heparin in men with unstable coronary artery disease. *Lancet* 1990;**336**:827–830.
27. Théroux P, *et al.* Aspirin, heparin, or both to treat acute unstable angina. *N Engl J Med* 1988;**319**:1105–1111.
28. Klimt C, *et al.* Persantine-Aspirin Reinfarction Study. Part II. Secondary prevention with persantine and aspirin. *J Am Coll Cardiol* 1986;**7**:251–269.
29. The Coronary Heart Drug Research Group. Aspirin in coronary heart disease. *Circulation* 1980;**62**(Suppl V):V59–V62.
30. The Persantine-Aspirin Reinfarction Study (PARIS) Research Group. Persantine and aspirin in coronary heart disease. *Circulation* 1980;**62**:449–462.
31. Antiplatelet Trialists' Collaboration. Collaborative overview of randomised trials of antiplatelet therapy — I. Prevention of death, myocardial infarction, and stroke by prolonged antiplatelet therapy in various categories of patients. *Br Med J* 1994;**308**:81–106.
32. Peto R, *et al.* Randomised trial of prophylactic aspirin in British male doctors. *Br Med J* 1988;**296**:313–316.
33. Steering Committee of the Physicians' Health Study Research Group. Final report on the aspirin component of the ongoing physicians' health study. *N Engl J Med* 1989;**321**(3):129–135.
34. Collaborative Group for the Primary Prevention Project. *L*ow-dose aspirin and vitamin E in people at cardiovascular risk: a randomised trial in general practice. *Lancet* 2001;**357**:89–95.
35. Hansson L, *et al.* Effects of intensive blood-pressure lowering and low-dose aspirin in patients with hypertension: principal results of the Hypertension Optimal Treatment (HOT) randomised trial. *Lancet* 1998;**351**:1755–1762.

36. Juul-Moller S, *et al.* Double-blind trial of aspirin in primary prevention of myocardial infarction in patients with stable chronic angina pectoris. *Lancet* 1992;**340**:1421–1425.
37. The Medical Research Council's General Practice Research Framework. Thrombosis prevention trial: randomised trial of low-intensity oral anticoagulation with warfarin and low-dose aspirin in the primary prevention of ischaemic heart disease in men at increased risk. *Lancet* 1998;**351**:233–241.
38. Ridker PM, *et al.* A randomized trial of low-dose aspirin in the primary prevention of cardiovascular disease in women. *N Engl J Med* 2005;**352**(13):1293–1304.
39. Juul-Moller S, *et al.* Double-blind trial of aspirin in primary prevention of myocardial infarction in patients with stable chronic angina pectoris. The Swedish Angina Pectoris Aspirin Trial (SAPAT) Group. *Lancet* 1992;**340**(8833):1421–1425.
40. Gruentzig AR, Senning A, Siegenthaler WE. Nonoperative dilatation of coronary-artery stenosis. *N Engl J Med* 1979;**301**:61–68.
41. Schwartz L, *et al.* Aspirin and dipyridamole in the prevention of restenosis after percutaneous transluminal coronary angioplasty. *N Engl J Med* 1988;**318**:1714–1719.
42. White CW, *et al.* Antiplatelet agents are effective in reducing the acute ischemic complications of angioplasty but do not prevent restenosis: results from the ticlopidine trial. *Coron Artery Dis* 1991;**2**:757–767.
43. Savage MP, *et al.* Effect of thromboxane A2 blockade on clinical outcome and restenosis after successful coronary angioplasty. Multi-Hospital Eastern Atlantic Restenosis Trial (M-HEART II). *Circulation* 1995;**92**:3194–3200.
44. Feldman M, Cryer B. Aspirin absorption rates and platelet inhibition times with 325-mg buffered aspirin tablets (chewed or swallowed intact) and with buffered aspirin solution. *Am J Cardiol* 1999;**84**:404–409.
45. Pedersen AK, FitzGerald GA. Dose-related kinetics of aspirin. Presystemic acetylation of platelet cyclooxygenase. *N Engl J Med* 1984;**311**:1206–1211.
46. Jimenez AH, *et al.* Rapidity and duration of platelet suppression by enteric-coated aspirin in healthy young men. *Am J Cardiol* 1992;**69**:258–262.
47. Buerke M., *et al.* Aspirin therapy: optimized platelet inhibition with different loading and maintenance doses. *Am Heart J* 1995;**130**:465–472.
48. Burch J, Stanford N, Majerus P. Inhibition of platelet prostaglandin synthase by oral aspirin. *J Clin Invest* 1979;**61**:314–319.
49. Patrignani P, Filabozzi P, Patrono C. Selective cumulative inhibition of platelet thromboxane production by low-dose aspirin in healthy subjects. *J Clin Invest* 1982;**69**:1366–1372.

50. Patrono C, *et al.* Clinical pharmacology of platelet cyclooxygenase inhibition. *Circulation* 1985;**72**(6):1177–1184.
51. Johnson E, *et al.* A metaregression analysis of the dose-response effect of aspirin on stroke. *Arch Intern Med* 1999;**159**:1248–1253.
52. Verheugt FWA. Differential dose effect of aspirin in the primary prevention of myocardial infarction [abst]. *J Am Coll Cardiol* 1998;**31**(Suppl A):352A.
53. Taylor DW, *et al.* Low-dose and high-dose acetylsalicylic acid for patients undergoing carotid endarterectomy: a ramdomised controlled trial. *Lancet* 1999;**353**:2179–2184.
54. Grotemeyer KH, Scharafinski HW, Husstedt IW. Two-year follow-up of aspirin responder and aspirin non-responder. A pilot-study including 180 post-stroke patients. *Thromb Res* 1993;**71**(5):397–403.
55. Eikelboom JW, *et al.* Aspirin-resistant thromboxane biosynthesis and the risk of myocardial infarction, stroke, or cardiovascular death in patients at high risk for cardiovascular events. *Circulation* 2002;**105**(14):1650–1655.
56. Gum PA, *et al.* Profile and prevalence of aspirin resistance in patients with cardiovascular disease. *Am J Cardiol* 2001;**88**(3):230–235.
57. Chen WH, *et al.* Aspirin resistance is associated with a high incidence of myonecrosis after non-urgent percutaneous coronary intervention despite clopidogrel pretreatment. *J Am Coll Cardiol* 2004;**43**(6):1122–1126.
58. Catella-Lawson F, *et al.* Cyclooxygenase inhibitors and the antiplatelet effects of aspirin. *N Engl J Med* 2001;**345**(25):1809–1817.
59. Pedersen AK, FitzGerald GA. Dose-related kinetics of aspirin. Presystemic acetylation of platelet cyclooxygenase. *N Engl J Med* 1984;**311**(19): 1206–1211.
60. Benedek IH, *et al.* Variability in the pharmacokinetics and pharmacodynamics of low dose aspirin in healthy male volunteers. *J Clin Pharmacol* 1995;**35**(12):1181–1186.
61. Patrono C, *et al.* Clinical pharmacology of platelet cyclooxygenase inhibition. *Circulation* 1985;**72**(6):1177–1184.
62. Capone ML, *et al.* Pharmacodynamic interaction of naproxen with low-dose aspirin in healthy subjects. *J Am Coll Cardiol* 2005;**45**(8):1295–301.
63. Derry S, Loke YK. Risk of gastrointestinal haemorrhage with long term use of aspirin: meta-analysis. *BMJ* 2000;**321**:1183–1187.
64. Weil J, *et al.* Prophylactic aspirin and risk of peptic ulcer bleeding. *Br Med J* 1995;**310**:827–830.
65. Hofteizer JW, *et al.* Comparison of the effects of regular and enteric coated aspirin on gastroduodenal mucosa of man. *Lancet* 1980;**2**:609–612.
66. Kelly J, *et al.* Risk of aspirin-associated major upper-gastrointestinal bleeding with enteric-coated or buffered product. *Lancet* 1996;**348**:1413–1416.

67. He J, *et al.* Aspirin and risk of hemorrhagic stroke: a meta-analysis of randomized controlled trials. *JAMA* 1998;**280**(22):1930–1935.
68. Gresele P, Momi S, Mezzasoma AM. NCX4016: a novel antithrombotic agent. *Dig Liver Dis* 2003;**35**(Suppl 2):S20–26.
69. Akaike T. Role of free radicals in viral pathogenesis and mutation. *Rev Med Virol* 2001;**11**(2):87–101.
70. Zhao M-L, Kim M-O, Morgello S, Lee SC. Expression of inducible nitric oxide synthase, interleukin-1 and caspase-1 in HIV-1 encephalitis. *J Neuroimmunol* 2001;**115**(1–2):182–191.
71. Stamler JS, Vaughan DE, Loscalzo J. *S*ynergistic disaggregation of platelets by tissue-type plasminogen activator, prostaglandin E1, and nitroglycerin. *Circ Res* 1989;**65**(3):796–804.
72. Loscalzo J. Nitric oxide insufficiency, platelet activation, and arterial thrombosis. *Circ Res* 2001;**88**(8):756–762.
73. Ignarro LJ, *et al.* Role of the arginine-nitric oxide pathway in the regulation of vascular smooth muscle cell proliferation. *Proc Natl Acad Sci USA* 2001;**98**(7):4202–4208.
74. Guzik TJ, Korbut R, Adamek-Guzik T. Nitric oxide and superoxide in inflammation and immune regulation. *J Physiol Pharmacol* 2003;**54**(4):469–487.
75. Moncada S, Palmer RM, Higgs EA. Nitric oxide: physiology, pathophysiology, and pharmacology. *Pharmacol Rev* 1991;**43**(2):109–142.
76. Ignarro LJ, *et al.* Endothelium-derived relaxing factor produced and released from artery and vein is nitric oxide. *Proc Natl Acad Sci USA* 1987;**84**(24):9265–9269.
77. Moncada S, Higgs A, Furchgott R. International Union of Pharmacology Nomenclature in Nitric Oxide Research. *Pharmacol Rev* 1997;**49**(2): 137–142.
78. Brunori M, *et al.* Nitric oxide and cellular respiration. *Cell Mol Life Sci* 1999;**56**(7–8):549–557.
79. Wiesinger H. Arginine metabolism and the synthesis of nitric oxide in the nervous system. *Prog Neurobiol* 2001;**64**(4):365–391.
80. Luo ZD, Cizkova D. The role of nitric oxide in nociception. *Curr Rev Pain* 2000;**4**(6):459–466.
81. Jourd'heuil D, Grisham MB, Granger DN. Nitric oxide and the gut. *Curr Gastroenterol Rep* 1999;**1**(5):384–388.
82. Holzmann A, *et al.* Inhibition of lung phosphodiesterase improves responsiveness to inhaled nitric oxide in isolated-perfused lungs from rats challenged with endotoxin. *Intensive Care Med* 2001;**27**(1):251–257.
83. Wallace JL, Ignarro LJ, Fiorucci S. Potential cardioprotective actions of no-releasing aspirin. *Nat Rev Drug Discov* 2002;**1**(5):375–382.

84. Wallace JL, *et al.* Anti-thrombotic effects of a nitric oxide-releasing, gastric-sparing aspirin derivative. *J Clin Invest* 1995;**96**(6):2711–2718.
85. Lechi C, *et al.* The antiplatelet effects of a new nitroderivative of acetylsalicylic acid — an *in vitro* study of inhibition on the early phase of platelet activation and on TXA2 production. *Thromb Haemost* 1996;**76**(5): 791–798.
86. Shukla N, *et al.* Nitric oxide donating aspirins: novel drugs for the treatment of saphenous vein graft failure. *Ann Thorac Surg* 2003;**75**(5):1437–1442.
87. Napoli C, *et al.* Effects of nitric oxide-releasing aspirin versus aspirin on restenosis in hypercholesterolemic mice. *Proc Natl Acad Sci USA* 2001;**98**(5):2860–2864.
88. Napoli C, *et al.* Efficacy and age-related effects of nitric oxide-releasing aspirin on experimental restenosis. *Proc Natl Acad Sci USA* 2002;**99**(3):1689–1694.
89. Rossoni G, *et al.* The nitroderivative of aspirin, NCX 4016, reduces infarct size caused by myocardial ischemia-reperfusion in the anesthetized rat. *J Pharmacol Exp Ther* 2001;**297**(1):380–387.
90. Fredduzzi S, *et al.* Nitro-aspirin (NCX4016) reduces brain damage induced by focal cerebral ischemia in the rat. *Neurosci Lett* 2001;**302**(2–3):121–124.
91. Dogne JM, *et al.* New trends in thromboxane and prostacyclin modulators. *Curr Med Chem* 2000;**7**(6):609–628.
92. Coleman RA, *et al.* Comparison of the actions of U-46619, a prostaglandin H2-analogue, with those of prostaglandin H2 and thromboxane A2 on some isolated smooth muscle preparations. *Br J Pharmacol* 1981;**73**(3):773–778.
93. Vermylen J, Deckmyn H. Thromboxane synthase inhibitors and receptor antagonists. *Cardiovasc Drugs Ther* 1992;**6**(1):29–33.
94. Minoguchi K, Adachi M. Thromboxane A2 synthase inhibitor and receptor antagonist. *Nippon Rinsho* 2001;**59**(10):1986–1991.
95. Patscheke H, Hornberger W, Zehender H. Pathophysiological role of thromboxane A2 and pharmacological approaches to its inhibition. *Z Kardiol* 1990;**79**(Suppl 3):151–154.
96. Patrono C. Biosynthesis and pharmacological modulation of thromboxane in humans. *Circulation* 1990;**81**(Suppl 1):I12–15; discussion I22–23.
97. Habib A, FitzGerald GA, MacLouf J. Phosphorylation of the thromboxane receptor alpha, the predominant isoform expressed in human platelets. *J Biol Chem* 1999;**274**(5):2645–2651.
98. Miggin SM, Kinsella BT. Expression and tissue distribution of the mRNAs encoding the human thromboxane A2 receptor (TP) alpha and beta isoforms. *Biochim Biophys Acta* 1998;**1425**(3):543–559.

99. Gomoll AW, Grover GI, Ogletree ML. Myocardial salvage efficacy of the thromboxane receptor antagonist ifetroban in ferrets and dogs. *J Cardiovasc Pharmacol* 1994;**24**(6):960–968.
100. Serruys PW, *et al.* Prevention of restenosis after percutaneous transluminal coronary angioplasty with thromboxane A2-receptor blockade. A randomized, double-blind, placebo-controlled trial. Coronary Artery Restenosis Prevention on Repeated Thromboxane-Antagonism Study (CARPORT). *Circulation* 1991;**84**(4):1568–1580.
101. Savage MP, *et al.* Effect of thromboxane A2 blockade on clinical outcome and restenosis after successful coronary angioplasty. Multi-Hospital Eastern Atlantic Restenosis Trial (M-HEART II). *Circulation* 1995;**92**(11): 3194–3200.
102. Belhassen L, *et al.* Improved endothelial function by the thromboxane A2 receptor antagonist S 18886 in patients with coronary artery disease treated with aspirin. *J Am Coll Cardiol* 2003;**41**(7):1198–1204.
103. Kariyazono H, *et al.* Evaluation of anti-platelet aggregatory effects of aspirin, cilostazol and ramatroban on platelet-rich plasma and whole blood. *Blood Coagul Fibrinolysis* 2004;**15**(2):157–167.
104. Ishizuka T, *et al.* Ramatroban (BAY u 3405): a novel dual antagonist of TXA2 receptor and CRTh2, a newly identified prostaglandin D2 receptor. *Cardiovasc Drug Rev* 2004;**22**(2):71–90.
105. Schenk JF, *et al.* Antiplatelet and anticoagulant effects of "HN-11 500," a selective thromboxane receptor antagonist. *Thromb Res* 2001;**103**(2):79–91.
106. Neri Serneri GG, *et al.* Picotamide, a combined inhibitor of thromboxane A2 synthase and receptor, reduces 2-year mortality in diabetics with peripheral arterial disease: the DAVID study. *Eur Heart J* 2004;**25**(20):1845–1852.
107. Sone H, *et al.* Acute effects of thromboxane dual blocker (KDI-792) on different portions of lower limb blood flow — a study using Doppler ultrasonography and laser Doppler flowmetry in type 2 diabetic patients. *Prostaglandins* 1997;**53**(6):395–409.
108. Guth BD, *et al.* Pharmacokinetics and pharmacodynamics of terbogrel, a combined thromboxane A2 receptor and synthase inhibitor, in healthy subjects. *Br J Clin Pharmacol* 2004;**58**(1):40–51.
109. Langleben D, *et al.* Effects of the thromboxane synthetase inhibitor and receptor antagonist terbogrel in patients with primary pulmonary hypertension. *Am Heart J* 2002;**143**(5):E4.
110. Galie N, Manes A, Branzi A. The new clinical trials on pharmacological treatment in pulmonary arterial hypertension. *Eur Respir J* 2002;**20**(4): 1037–1049.

111. Randomized trial of ridogrel, a combined thromboxane A2 synthase inhibitor and thromboxane A2/prostaglandin endoperoxide receptor antagonist, versus aspirin as adjunct to thrombolysis in patients with acute myocardial infarction. The Ridogrel Versus Aspirin Patency Trial (RAPT). *Circulation* 1994;**89**(2):588–595.
112. Tytgat GN, *et al.* Efficacy and safety of oral ridogrel in the treatment of ulcerative colitis: two multicentre, randomized, double-blind studies. *Aliment Pharmacol Ther* 2002;**16**(1):87–99.
113. Carty E, *et al.* Thromboxane synthase immunohistochemistry in inflammatory bowel disease. *J Clin Pathol* 2002;**55**(5):367–70.
114. Final report on the aspirin component of the ongoing Physicians' Health Study. Steering Committee of the Physicians' Health Study Research Group. *N Engl J Med* 1989;**321**(3):129–135.
115. Peto R, *et al.* Randomised trial of prophylactic daily aspirin in British male doctors. *Br Med J (Clin Res Ed)* 1988;**296**(6618):313–316.
116. Thrombosis prevention trial: randomised trial of low-intensity oral anticoagulation with warfarin and low-dose aspirin in the primary prevention of ischaemic heart disease in men at increased risk. The Medical Research Council's General Practice Research Framework. *Lancet* 1998;**351**(9098):233–241.
117. Hansson L, *et al.* Effects of intensive blood-pressure lowering and low-dose aspirin in patients with hypertension: principal results of the Hypertension Optimal Treatment (HOT) randomised trial. HOT Study Group. *Lancet* 1998. 351(9118):1755–1762.
118. de Gaetano G. Low-dose aspirin and vitamin E in people at cardiovascular risk: a randomised trial in general practice. Collaborative Group of the Primary Prevention Project. *Lancet* 2001;**357**(9250):89–95.
119. Tyler HM, Saxton CA, Parry MJ, Administration to man of UK-37,248-01, a selective inhibitor of thromboxane synthetase. *Lancet* 1981;**1**(8221): 629–632.
120. Vermylen J, *et al.* Thromboxane synthetase inhibition as antithrombotic strategy. *Lancet* 1981;**1**(8229):1073–1075.
121. FitzGerald GA, *et al.* Endogenous prostacyclin biosynthesis and platelet function during selective inhibition of thromboxane synthase in man. *J Clin Invest* 1983;**72**(4):1336–1343.
122. Patrignani P, *et al.* Differential effects of dazoxiben, a selective thromboxane-synthase inhibitor, on platelet and renal prostaglandin-endoperoxide metabolism. *J Pharmacol Exp Ther* 1984;**228**(2):472–477.

123. MacNab MW, *et al.* The effects of a new thromboxane synthetase inhibitor, CGS-13080, in man. *J Clin Pharmacol* 1984;**24**(2–3):76–83.
124. Mohrland JS, Vander Lugt JT, Lakings DB, Multiple dose trial of the thromboxane synthase inhibitor furegrelate in normal subjects. *Eur J Clin Pharmacol* 1990;**38**(5):485–488.
125. Reuben SR, *et al.* Effects of dazoxiben on exercise performance in chronic stable angina. *Br J Clin Pharmacol* 1983;**15**(Suppl 1):83S-86S.
126. Hendra T, *et al.* Dazoxiben in stable angina. *Lancet* 1983;**1**(8332):1041.
127. Kiff PS, *et al.* Haemodynamic and metabolic effects of dazoxiben at rest and during atrial pacing. *Br J Clin Pharmacol*, 1983;**15**(Suppl 1):73S–77S.
128. Hutton I, *et al.,* Effects of dazoxiben on transcardiac thromboxane levels and haemodynamics in coronary heart disease. *Br J Clin Pharmacol* 1983;**15**(Suppl 1):79S-82S.
129. Thaulow E, Dale J, Myhre E. Effects of a selective thromboxane synthetase inhibitor, dazoxiben, and of acetylsalicylic acid on myocardial ischemia in patients with coronary artery disease. *Am J Cardiol* 1984;**53**(9):1255–1258.
130. Reilly IA, *et al.* Increased thromboxane biosynthesis in a human preparation of platelet activation: biochemical and functional consequences of selective inhibition of thromboxane synthase. *Circulation* 1986;**73**(6):1300–1309.
131. He GW, Yang CQ. Inhibition of vasoconstriction by the thromboxane A2 antagonist GR32191B in the human radial artery. *Br J Clin Pharmacol* 1999;**48**(2):207–215.
132. Matsuno H, *et al.* Pharmacokinetic and pharmacodynamic properties of a new thromboxane receptor antagonist (Z-335) after single and multiple oral administrations to healthy volunteers. *J Clin Pharmacol* 2002;**42**(7):782–790.
133. Ghuysen A, *et al.* Pharmacological profile and therapeutic potential of BM-573, a combined thromboxane receptor antagonist and synthase inhibitor. *Cardiovasc Drug Rev* 2005;**23**(1):1–14.

3 Glycoprotein IIb/IIIa Inhibitors

Sam J. Lehman, Derek P. Chew and Harvey D. White

Introduction

Platelet aggregation in acute coronary syndromes and percutaneous coronary intervention

Angiographic and pathological studies have demonstrated the critical role of thrombus formation and platelet aggregation in acute coronary syndromes.[1–3] Occlusive thrombus in coronary arteries begins with deposition of platelets on a ruptured or eroded atherosclerotic plaque.[4] Platelet adherence is mediated by the interaction of receptors on the platelet surface with subendothelial proteins. The first layer of adherent platelets probably has little effect on blood flow. It is the recruitment of additional layers of platelets and platelet aggregation that pose the greatest risk of platelet-thrombus formation and occlusion of the coronary artery.[5] The glycoprotein (GP) IIb/IIIa receptor plays a pivotal role in this process of platelet aggregation.[6,7] It is on this basis that antagonists to the platelet GP IIb/IIIa receptors have been developed for use in cardiovascular disease. They have been evaluated in the two situations that involve the highest degree of coronary platelet aggregation. These are acute coronary syndromes and percutaneous coronary interventions.

Glycoprotein IIb/IIIa in platelet physiology

There are three phases in the response of platelets to tissue injury. The first is adhesion. Platelets adhere to exposed collagen, von Willebrand factor (vWf), and fibrinogen by specific cell receptors. Adherent platelets can then be activated by thrombin, collagen, thromboxane, serotonin, epinephrine, and adenosine diphosphate (ADP) in the second phase. Activated platelets degranulate and secrete chemotaxins, clotting factors and vasoconstrictors. This promotes thrombin generation, vasospasm, and additional platelet accumulation.

The third phase of platelet response is aggregation. GP IIb/IIIa is the most abundant receptor on the surface of the platelet and is an important pathway for platelet aggregation.[6] There are approximately 50,000 GP IIb/IIIa receptors on each platelet. The GP IIb/IIIa receptor is a member of the integrin family of adhesion molecules. These are calcium dependent heterodimers, composed of an α- and a β-subunit. In the resting state, the receptor has a low affinity for fibrinogen.[8] When the platelet becomes activated, however, the GP IIb/IIIa receptor develops a high affinity for the fibrinogen molecule (Fig. 1). Fibrinogen is a bivalent molecule with binding sites for the GP IIb/IIIa receptor at both ends, allowing a bridge to be formed between two adjacent platelets.[9]

GP IIb/IIIa receptor expression and function are dynamic and responsive to the platelets internal state of activation (inside-to-outside signaling).[10] Platelet activation results in increased receptor expression and binding affinity. The platelets internal microenvironment is also influenced by ligand binding to the GP IIb/IIIa receptor. This outside-to-inside

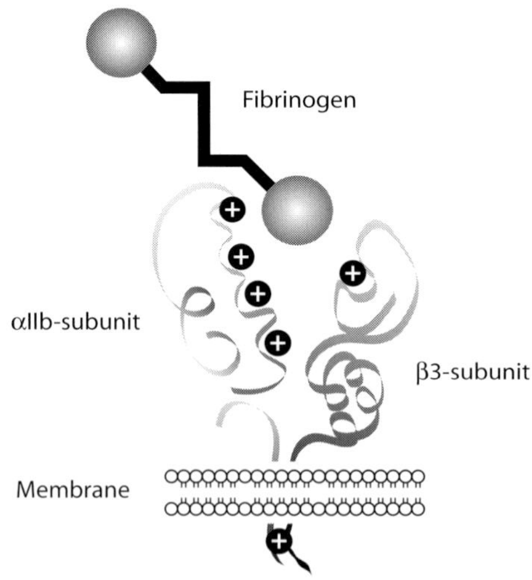

Fig. 1. Fibrinogen binding to the GP IIb/IIIa receptor.

signaling through the activated GP IIb/IIIa receptor provokes an array of intracellular signals.[11,12]

Activated platelets in the thrombus have catalytic surfaces on which thrombin can be generated, leading to fibrin deposition and further platelet activation and adhesion.

Heterogeneity in clinical trial data

The trials of aspirin and the thienopyridine clopidogrel in stable angina and acute coronary syndromes have been universally positive.[13–15] The use of aspirin and thienopyridines has also become the standard of care in percutaneous coronary intervention (PCI). The striking feature of the GP IIb/IIIa inhibitor data is the heterogeneity. The oral agents have shown a trend towards increased mortality despite a number of agents and dosing regimens.[16] Data for the intravenous agents is positive only in selected circumstances. Interpretation of the data requires consideration of a number of factors.

Dosing appears critically important to the clinical outcomes with GP IIb/IIIa inhibitors. It appears from both animal and early dose finding data in humans that the critical level of receptor blockade is 80%.[17–19] Low levels of synthetic antagonists appear to activate quiescent receptors. This cannot only increase the population of high-affinity receptors available for binding, but also increase the expression of inflammatory signaling adhesion molecules. Therefore, a pro-aggregatory state may result from subtherapeutic dosing of GP IIb/IIIa inhibitors.[20] The GOLD (AU-Assessing Ultegra) study demonstrated the level of platelet inhibition with GP IIb/IIIa inhibitors was an independent predictor for death and ischemic complications after PCI (Fig. 2).[21]

Timing of GP IIb/IIIa inhibition is important for efficacy and safety. The aim is to use these agents at the time of maximum platelet aggregation. Significant disruption of the coronary plaque occurs at the time of either balloon angioplasty or intra-coronary stent implantation. It is not surprising that the maximum effectiveness of the use of intravenous GP IIb/IIIa inhibitors is around this time. While a benefit for tirofiban and eptifibatide has been shown in patients with acute coronary syndromes treated conservatively, this has not been the case with abciximab.

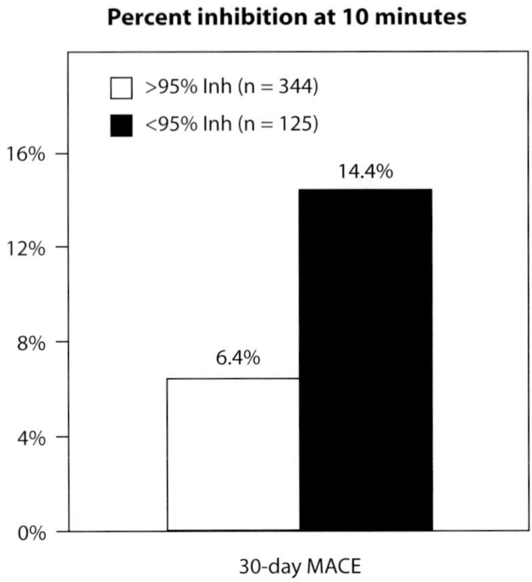

Fig. 2. Data from the GOLD study demonstrating a correlation between level of GP IIb/IIIa inhibition and clinical outcomes from percutaneous coronary intervention. Major Cardiac Events (MACE) is a composite of death, myocardial infarction, and urgent target vessel revascularization.[21]

The third factor critical to the use of GP IIb/IIIa inhibitors is adequate risk stratification. Increased troponin levels are associated with platelet emboli and micro-infarction and predict a more unstable milieu at the coronary plaque. In the acute coronary syndrome trials, there have been consistently greater benefits with these agents in troponin positive patients. Subgroups of patients in some trials who were troponin negative have had increased mortality rates. Troponin is not the only marker of increased risk and therefore benefit from GP IIb/IIIa use. Subgroup analysis from the Randomized Placebo-Controlled Trial of Abciximab Before and During Coronary Intervention in Refractory Unstable Angina (CAPTURE) trial revealed the inflammatory marker CD 40 ligand to be a powerful predictor of risk and subsequent benefit from abciximab therapy.[22]

The additional cost, heterogenous and complex data, as well as a perceived increase in major bleeding risk has delayed the widespread clinical uptake of these agents. Intravenous GP IIb/IIIa inhibitor therapy has become the standard of care for patients undergoing high risk PCI. The situation for patients at lower risk of ischemic complications of these procedures, who have been pre-treated with aspirin and clopidogrel is less clear.

Abciximab

A murine monoclonal antibody directed at the GP IIb/IIIa receptor (7E3) was first described by Coller.[23,24] In order to reduce immunogenicity to humans, the murine 7E3 was redesigned as a part-murine, part-human chimeric Fab fragment using recombinant techniques. This combined product (c7E3, abciximab) contains the heavy and light chain variable regions from the murine antibody attached to the constant regions of human antibody.

Abciximab has a short half-life of around 30 minutes.[25] For this reason, the bolus dose must be followed with an infusion. The drug is avidly, but reversibly, bound to platelets and the antiplatelet effect lasts much longer. Bleeding time returns to normal in 12 hours, and platelet aggregation in response to adenosine diphosphate (ADP) is normal in one to two days in most people. Abciximab is cleared from the circulation by the reticuloendothelial system. The actions of abciximab can be overcome by platelet transfusion.

Thrombocytopenia within 24 hours of abciximab administration is well described. The potential of abciximab to stimulate antibodies has raised concerns regarding allergic reactions on readminstration. In a prospective review of 550 patients receiving a second or third dose of abciximab at least seven days after the first treatment, there were no cases of allergic complications.[26]

Trials of abciximab in PCI have consistently shown an increase in minor, but not major bleeding episodes. One of the most feared complications of antiplatelet therapy is hemorrhagic stroke. A meta-analysis of patients undergoing percutaneous coronary intervention did not show an increase in stroke.[27–30] There was however, a non-significant trend towards an increase in intracranial bleeding with combined use of abciximab and standard dose heparin compared with a lower dose heparin regimen. Other bleeding complications are also reduced by a low dose heparin compared with standard dose heparin use.

planned.[28] Patients with refractory unstable angina were treated with heparin and nitrates and underwent coronary angiography. After angiography, patients received a randomly assigned infusion of abciximab or placebo for 18 to 24 hours before PCI, continuing until one hour post-procedure. Both before and during PCI, abciximab therapy was associated with a lower rate of myocardial infarction. This benefit did not persist at six months. Major bleeding was infrequent, but occurred more often with abciximab than with placebo. The lower rate of peri-procedural myocardial infarction with abciximab may have been related to the higher rate of thrombus resolution noted with abciximab therapy in the angiographic substudy.[38] The benefits of abciximab therapy were greater if high risk features were present (complex lesion, troponin elevation, or elevated CD 40 ligand).[22,39]

Abciximab has known cross-reactivity with the $\alpha v\beta 3$ receptor, expressed mostly on endothelial and smooth muscle cells. This has prompted studies of abciximab on restenosis. Angiographic follow-up in two studies did not show a reduction in restenosis with abciximab therapy.[40,41] In the setting of diabetes, however, the ISAR-SWEET trial demonstrated a reduction in the rate of bare metal stent angiographic restenosis at a median of seven months (29% versus 38%, $p = 0.01$).[36]

The Effect of Glycoprotein IIb/IIIa Receptor Blocker Abciximab on Outcome in Patients with Acute Coronary Syndromes without Early Coronary Revascularization (GUSTO 4-ACS) trial examined the use of abciximab in patients with unstable angina, where PCI was not planned.[42] There was no benefit to the use of abciximab. Those with body weight less than 75 kilograms, negative baseline troponin, or elevated baseline C-reactive protein had increased mortality in association with abciximab. The lack of benefit with abciximab persisted at one year.[43]

Abciximab in ST segment elevation myocardial infarction

GP IIb/IIIa inhibitors do not appear incrementally beneficial when combined with thrombolytic agents in the treatment of ST segment elevation myocardial infarction.[44] An increased rate of intracerebral hemorrhage has been noted with abciximab and fibrinolysis in the elderly.[45,46]

Abciximab is beneficial in conjunction with primary angioplasty for the treatment of ST segment elevation myocardial infarction. Two trials have revealed primary angioplasty with abciximab decreased the incidence of death, reinfarction or urgent TVR.[47,48] This occurred at a cost of increased major bleeding episodes. Several non-randomized studies have shown that this benefit extends to the subgroup in cardiogenic shock.[49]

The Comparison of Angioplasty with Stenting, with or without Abciximab, in Acute Myocardial Infarction (CADILLAC) trial examined the use of balloon angioplasty, stenting and abciximab in the management of acute ST segment elevation myocardial infarction.[50] Patients presenting with acute myocardial infarction were randomized to balloon angioplasty, balloon angioplasty plus abciximab, stenting, or stenting plus abciximab. The major benefits in this trial were seen with the use of stents, regardless of the use of abciximab.

An important question is when to give abciximab in the setting of ST segment elevation myocardial infarction. Most trials have given the drug just prior to angioplasty. The Platelet Glycoprotein IIb/IIIa Inhibition with Coronary Stenting for Acute Myocardial Infarction (ADMIRAL) trial started abciximab earlier, and noted an improvement in pre-procedural flow and subsequent clinical outcome, particularly when it was started in the ambulance or emergency department.[51] A meta-analysis reviewing the six trials that have examined this issue found a trend towards reduction in mortality with early administration of abciximab, but this did not reach statistical significance (odds ratio 0.72, confidence interval, 0.37–1.40, $p = 0.42$).[52]

Small Molecule GP IIb/IIIa Inhibitors

There have been three non-antibody intravenous inhibitors of the GP IIb/IIIa receptor tested in phase III clinical trials. These molecules have potential clinical advantages of shorter biological half-life and no concern regarding immunogenicity. This alleviates the concern regarding re-adminstration.

Tirofiban is a tyrosine derivative, an active antagonist against the RGD binding site of the GP IIb/IIIa receptor.[53] Tirofiban has a half-life of two hours and is predominantly cleared renally. Eptifibatide is a cyclic heptapeptide modeled on the structure of barbourin, an inhibitor of GP IIb/IIIa found in the Southeastern pygmy rattlesnake. It has a plasma half-life of 150 minutes and is predominantly cleared renally. The level of platelet inhibition is dose dependent and related to plasma concentrations. Lamifiban is a renally excreted, non-peptide inhibitor of the GP IIb/IIIa receptor.

The bulk of clinical trial work with small molecule GP IIb/IIIa inhibitors is in the setting of Unstable Angina/Non-ST Segment Elevation Myocardial Infarction (UA/NSTEMI). There is evidence that tirofiban use in addition to heparin reduces ischemic complications in patients with unstable angina/NSTEMI, whether treated conservatively or interventionally.[54] The benefits seem to be greatest in those patients at highest risk for ischemic complications. The Comparison of Early Invasive and Conservative Strategies in Patients with Unstable Coronary Syndromes Treated with the Glycoprotein IIb/IIIa Inhibitor Tirofiban (TACTICS TIMI-18) trial supported the early use of tirofiban in conjunction with an early invasive strategy for the management of UA/NSTEMI.[55] In the Platelet Receptor Inhibition in Ischemic Syndrome Management (PRISM) study, benefit with the use of tirofiban was confined to the subset of patients who had elevated troponin levels.[56]

The issue of tirofiban use without heparin was examined in the PRISM-PLUS[57] study. In this trial, the tirofiban only group was discontinued prematurely due to an excess seven-day mortality. On this basis, tirofiban is not recommended for use without anticoagulation.

The Platelet Glycoprotein IIb/IIIa in Unstable Angina: Receptor Suppression using Integrilin Therapy (PURSUIT) trial was a large multinational study of the use of eptifibatide in addition to heparin in acute coronary syndromes.[58] There was a statistically significant reduction in the composite endpoint among patients receiving eptifibatide compared with placebo (15.7% versus 14.2%, $p = 0.04$). The benefit of eptifibatide was present regardless of invasive or conservative management, but greater in those who received coronary revascularization.

The Platelet IIb/IIIa Antagonism for the Reduction of Acute Coronary Syndrome Events in a Global Organization Network (PARAGON) A trial showed a benefit to the addition of lamifiban to aspirin and heparin in the management of UA/NSTEMI.[59] The PARAGON B trial did not show an overall benefit of lamifiban in addition to aspirin and heparin for NSTEMI.

There was a reduction in the primary composite endpoint in those who were troponin positive.[60]

A meta-analysis comparing the trials of all small molecule agents in patients not intended to undergo PCI revealed a 9% reduction in the odds of death or myocardial infarction.[61] This benefit was not seen in troponin negative women.

The small molecule GP IIb/IIIa inhibitors have been studied in the setting of elective or urgent PCI. The Additive Value of Tirofiban Administered with the High-Dose Bolus in the Prevention of Ischemic Complications During High-Risk Coronary Angioplasty (ADVANCE) study showed tirofiban to reduce ischemic complications, but did not reduce target vessel revascularization or death.[62] Eptifibatide has also been shown to have benefits in PCI. The Integrilin to Minimize Platelet Aggregation and Coronary Thrombosis (IMPACT) II trial demonstrated a significant reduction in early abrupt closure and 30-day ischemic events in the lower dose group.[63] The benefits were non-significant in the higher dose group. No difference was found in the incidence of major bleeding episodes. A novel double bolus dosing administration of eptifibatide in the Eptifibatide in Planned Coronary Stent Implantation (ESPRIT) trial reduced the rates of early ischemic complications of coronary stenting (6.6% versus 10.5%, $p = 0.0015$).[64]

The small molecule GP IIb/IIIa inhibitors have not been studied as extensively as abciximab in the setting of primary angioplasty. The Tirofiban in Myocardial Infarction Evaluation (ON TIME) trial examined the use of tirofiban use prior to the catheterization laboratory in primary angioplasty for acute myocardial infarction.[65] There was no benefit in TIMI flow post-PCI and, at one year, there was no difference in rate of death or recurrent infarct (7.0% versus 7.0%, $p = 0.99$).

Tirofiban use in the setting of non-reperfused infarcts was examined in the Safety and Efficacy of Subcutaneous Enoxaparin versus Intravenous Unfractionated Heparin and Tirofiban versus Placebo in the Treatment of Acute ST-Segment Elevation Myocardial Infarction Patients Ineligible for Reperfusion (TETAMI) trial.[66] There were similar results with the enoxaparin and unfractionated heparin. The addition of tirofiban did not add benefit to these regimens (odds ratio 1.02, 95% confidence interval 0.75 to 1.38).

Oral GP IIb/IIIa Inhibitors

The success of the intravenous small molecule GP IIb/IIIa inhibitors in acute coronary syndromes and percutaneous coronary interventions prompted development of oral forms. Several oral GP IIb/IIIa inhibitors have undergone clinical trials. These agents are prodrugs, converted to active metabolites in the liver.

There are several reasons for expecting positive outcomes with chronic inhibition of the GP IIb/IIIa receptor. Firstly, platelet activation is known to persist following acute coronary syndromes. There is also an association between spontaneous platelet aggregation and mortality following myocardial infarction.[67] A meta-analysis of the four largest trials of oral GP IIb/IIIa inhibitor therapy included 33,326 patients who were followed-up for more than 30 days.[16] Therapy with these agents increased mortality at three and six months (1.7% versus 1.3%, odds ratio 1.37, 95% confidence interval 1.13 to 1.66). There was also a significant increase in major bleeding (4% versus 2.4%, odds ratio 1.74), and urgent revascularization (2.8% versus 3.6%, odds ratio 0.77) (Fig. 3).

The Evaluation of Oral Xemilofiban in Controlling Thrombotic Events (EXCITE) trial compared xemilofiban (10 or 20 mg, three times daily for

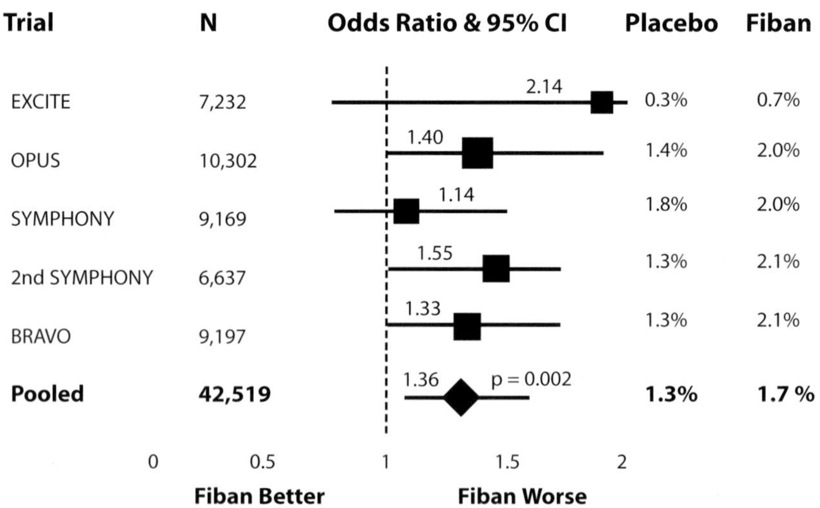

Fig. 3. Meta-analysis of mortality from the five large trials of oral GP IIb/IIIa inhibitors.[16]

two weeks and followed by daily for two weeks) with placebo in 7232 patients undergoing PCI.[68] At 30 days, there was a statistically significant increase in mortality in the xemilofiban group, with a non-significant reduction in MI. The Orbofiban in Patients with Unstable Coronary Syndromes (OPUS TIMI-16) trial randomized 10,302 patients with acute coronary syndromes to ether orbofiban 50 mg twice daily for six months or orbofiban 50 mg twice daily for 30 days followed by 30 mg twice daily for five months or placebo.[69] The study was terminated prematurely due to an excess 30-day mortality in the orbofiban treated groups. The Sibrafiban versus Aspirin to Yield Maximum Protection from Ischemic Heart Events Post-Acute Coronary Syndromes (SYMPHONY) and second SYMPHONY trials studied sibrafiban in acute coronary syndromes.[70,71] The SYMPHONY trial failed to demonstrate a reduction in ischemic endpoints. There was an excess mortality in the sibrafiban groups at 90 days in the second SYMPHONY trial. The Blockade of the Glycoprotein IIb/IIIa Receptor to Avoid Vascular Occlusion (BRAVO) trial examined the combined use of aspirin and lotrafiban in patients with a variety of vascular disease.[72] This included coronary, cerebrovascular, and peripheral vascular disease. The study was again terminated prematurely due to an excess mortality in the active treatment group.

There have been a number of proposed theories regarding the negative trial results of the oral GP IIb/IIIa inhibitors.[73] It may be that the benefits of GP IIb/IIIa inhibition are only present in the setting of co-existent antithrombin therapy. The oral agents may also act as partial agonists at the GP IIb/IIIa receptor. This may enhance inflammation within the vascular wall. Pharmacokinetic issues with oral formulations may lead to inadequate receptor inhibition during a 24-hour period. There are also possible mechanisms unrelated to platelet activity. Cardiomyocyte apoptosis mediated by caspase-3 has been demonstrated in animal models with the RDG peptides.[74] Despite these theories, the exact mechanism of loss of efficacy with the oral formulations is unknown.

New Trials of GP IIb/IIIa Inhibitors

The Acute Catheterization and Urgent Intervention Triage Strategy (ACUITY) trial is a large multinational trial of acute coronary syndrome (ACS) patients assigned to an early invasive management strategy.[75] Patients with moderate to high risk ACS are randomized to unfractionated heparin or enoxaparin plus GP IIb/IIIa inhibitors; or bivalirudin plus GP IIb/IIIa inhibitors; or bivalirudin plus provisional use of GP IIb/IIIa inhibitors. This trial will provide important information regarding the use of bivalirudin, and the necessity and optimal timing of additional GP IIb/IIIa inhibitors in ACS managed invasively.

The demonstrated inferiority of tirofiban compared with abciximab therapy in TARGET may have been due to an underdosing of the bolus. The Tirofiban Novel Dosing versus Abciximab with Evaluation of Clopidogrel and Inhibition of Thrombin (TENACITY) trial used a higher bolus dose of tirofiban than in TARGET and compared it head to head with abciximab. Intermediate to high risk patients received aspirin and clopidogrel 600 mg and were randomized on an intent to stent basis. They were randomized to either tirofiban (with either heparin or bivalirudin) or abciximab (with either heparin or bivalirudin). This study was terminated early due to lack of funding.

The Early Glycoprotein IIb/IIIa Inhibition in Non-ST-Segment Elevation Acute Coronary Syndrome (EARLY-ACS) trial will examine the role of early administration of eptifibatide with aspirin and heparin or enoxaparin in high risk NSTEMI. Patients in this study will be managed with an early invasive strategy.

Summary/Conclusions

There is a consistent benefit with GP IIb/IIIa inhibitor use in the setting of urgent or elective coronary PCI. There is also a consistent benefit of small molecule GP IIb/IIIa inhibitors in the setting of high risk unstable angina, treated either conservatively or interventionally. Benefit seems to be correlated with clinical and biochemical markers of ischemic risk. The results of ongoing trials will provide important information regarding the optimal use of these agents in acute coronary syndromes. The oral GP IIb/IIIa inhibitors are not currently marketed. Significant advances in the understanding of these agents are required before further clinical trials are undertaken.

Summary Box

The Role of GP IIb/IIIa Receptor in Acute Coronary Syndromes

- Platelet aggregation and thrombus formation are critical mechanisms in the acute coronary syndromes
- The GP IIb/IIIa receptor is a member of the integrin family, with binding sites for the fibrinogen molecule
- GP IIb/IIIa receptor plays a pivotal role in platelet aggregation
- Antagonists to the GP IIb/IIIa receptor have become important tools in acute coronary syndromes and percutaneous coronary intervention

Abciximab

- Abciximab is a part-murine, part-human chimeric Fab fragment against the GP IIb/IIIa receptor
- Platelet monitoring is important with abciximab therapy due to an association with thrombocytopenia
- Abciximab was superior to tirofiban in patients undergoing PCI in the TARGET trial
- Patients with unstable angina who did not receive PCI did not benefit from abciximab in the GUSTO 4-ACS trial

Small Molecule Inhibitors of GP IIb/IIIa Receptor

- Tirofiban and Eptifibatide have demonstrated efficacy in unstable angina, regardless of invasive or conservative management
- The benefits of these agents are greatest in those with unstable angina at high risk of ischemic complications
- Serum troponin levels are a useful predictor of risk

Oral GP IIb/IIIa Receptor Inhibitors

- A meta-analysis of the four largest trials of oral GP IIb/IIIa receptor inhibitors demonstrated increased mortality
- These agents have also been associated with an increase in major bleeding and urgent revascularization
- There are a number of proposed theories regarding the lack of efficacy of these agents

References

1. Stein B, Fuster V, Halperin JL, *et al.* Antithrombotic therapy in cardiac disease. An emerging approach based on pathogenesis and risk. *Circulation* 1989;**80**(6):1501–1513.
2. Fuster V, Lewis A. Conner Memorial Lecture. Mechanisms leading to myocardial infarction: insights from studies of vascular biology. *Circulation* 1994;**90**(4):2126–2146.
3. Mizuno K. Angioscopic examination of the coronary arteries: what have we learned? *Heart Dis Stroke* 1992;**1**(5):320–324.
4. Davies MJ. A macro and micro view of coronary vascular insult in ischemic heart disease. *Circulation* 1990;**82**(3 Suppl):II38–II46.
5. Fuster V, Badimon L, Badimon JJ, *et al.* The pathogenesis of coronary artery disease and the acute coronary syndromes (2). *N Engl J Med* 1992;**326**(5):310–318.
6. Cox D, Aoki T, Seki J, *et al.* The pharmacology of the integrins. *Med Res Rev* 1994;**14**(2):195–228.
7. Lefkovits J, Topol EJ. Platelet glycoprotein IIb/IIIa receptor antagonists in coronary artery disease. *Eur Heart J* 1996;**17**(1):9–18.
8. Cierniewski CS, Byzova T, Papierak M, *et al.* Peptide ligands can bind to distinct sites in integrin alpha IIb beta3 and elicit different functional responses. *J Biol Chem* 1999;**274**(24):16923–16932.
9. Plow EF, D'Souza SE, Ginsberg MH. Ligand binding to GPIIb-IIIa: a status report. *Semin Thromb Hemost* 1992;**18**(3):324–332.
10. Shattil SJ, Ginsberg MH. Integrin signaling in vascular biology. *J Clin Invest* 1997;**100**(11 Suppl):S91–95.
11. Rybak ME, Renzulli LA. Ligand inhibition of the platelet glycoprotein IIb-IIIa complex function as a calcium channel in liposomes. *J Biol Chem* 1989;**264**(25):14617–14620.
12. Du XP, Plow EF, Frelinger ALd, *et al.* Ligands "activate" integrin alpha IIb beta 3 (platelet GPIIb-IIIa). *Cell* 1991;**65**(3):409–416.
13. ISIS-2 (Second International Study of Infarct Survival) Collaborative Group. Randomized trial of intravenous streptokinase, oral aspirin, both, or neither among 17,187 cases of suspected acute myocardial infarction: ISIS-2. *Lancet* 1988;**2**(8607):349–360.
14. Cairns JA, Gent M, Singer J, *et al.* Aspirin, sulfinpyrazone, or both in unstable angina. Results of a Canadian multicenter trial. *N Engl J Med* 1985;**313**(22):1369–1375.

15. Antithrombotic Trialists' Collaboration. Collaborative meta-analysis of randomized trials of antiplatelet therapy for prevention of death, myocardial infarction, and stroke in high risk patients. *BMJ* 2002;**324**(7329):71–86.
16. Chew DP, Bhatt DL, Sapp S, *et al.* Increased mortality with oral platelet glycoprotein IIb/IIIa antagonists: a meta-analysis of phase III multicenter randomized trials. *Circulation* 2001;**103**(2):201–206.
17. Coller BS, Folts JD, Smith SR, *et al.* Abolition of *in vivo* platelet thrombus formation in primates with monoclonal antibodies to the platelet GPIIb/IIIa receptor. Correlation with bleeding time, platelet aggregation, and blockade of GPIIb/IIIa receptors. *Circulation* 1989;**80**(6):1766–1774.
18. Peter K, Straub A, Kohler B, *et al.* Platelet activation as a potential mechanism of GP IIb/IIIa inhibitor-induced thrombocytopenia. *Am J Cardiol* 1999;**84**(5):519–524.
19. Gawaz M, Ruf A, Neumann FJ, *et al.* Effect of glycoprotein IIb-IIIa receptor antagonism on platelet membrane glycoproteins after coronary stent placement. *Thromb Haemost* 1998;**80**(6):994–1001.
20. Peter K, Schwarz M, Ylanne J, *et al.* Induction of fibrinogen binding and platelet aggregation as a potential intrinsic property of various glycoprotein IIb/IIIa inhibitors. *Blood* 1998;**92**(9):3240–3249.
21. Steinhubl SR, Talley JD, Braden GA, *et al.* Point-of-care measured platelet inhibition correlates with a reduced risk of an adverse cardiac event after percutaneous coronary intervention: results of the GOLD (AU-Assessing Ultegra) multicenter study. *Circulation* 2001;**103**(21):2572–2578.
22. Heeschen C, Dimmeler S, Hamm CW, *et al.* Soluble CD40 ligand in acute coronary syndromes. *N Engl J Med* 2003;**348**(12):1104–1111.
23. Coller BS, Peerschke EI, Scudder LE, *et al.* A murine monoclonal antibody that completely blocks the binding of fibrinogen to platelets produces a thrombasthenic-like state in normal platelets and binds to glycoproteins IIb and/or IIIa. *J Clin Invest* 1983;**72**(1):325–338.
24. Coller BS. A new murine monoclonal antibody reports an activation-dependent change in the conformation and/or microenvironment of the platelet glycoprotein IIb/IIIa complex. *J Clin Invest* 1985;**76**(1):101–108.
25. Faulds D, Sorkin EM. Abciximab (c7E3 Fab). A review of its pharmacology and therapeutic potential in ischemic heart disease. *Drugs* 1994;**48**(4):583–598.
26. Tcheng JE, Kereiakes DJ, Lincoff AM, *et al.* Abciximab readministration: results of the ReoPro Readministration Registry. *Circulation* 2001;**104**(8):870–875.

27. The EPIC Investigation. Use of a monoclonal antibody directed against the platelet glycoprotein IIb/IIIa receptor in high-risk coronary angioplasty. *N Engl J Med* 1994;**330**(14):956–961.
28. The CAPTURE Investigators. Randomized placebo-controlled trial of abciximab before and during coronary intervention in refractory unstable angina: the CAPTURE Study. *Lancet* 1997;**349**(9063):1429–1435.
29. The EPILOG Investigators. Platelet glycoprotein IIb/IIIa receptor blockade and low-dose heparin during percutaneous coronary revascularization. *N Engl J Med* 1997;**336**(24):1689–1696.
30. Akkerhuis KM, Deckers JW, Lincoff AM, *et al.* Risk of stroke associated with abciximab among patients undergoing percutaneous coronary intervention. *JAMA* 2001;**286**(1):78–82.
31. Topol EJ, Lincoff AM, Kereiakes DJ, *et al.* Multi-year follow-up of abciximab therapy in three randomized, placebo-controlled trials of percutaneous coronary revascularization. *Am J Med* 2002;**113**(1):1–6.
32. Topol EJ, Ferguson JJ, Weisman HF, *et al.* Long-term protection from myocardial ischemic events in a randomized trial of brief integrin beta3 blockade with percutaneous coronary intervention. EPIC Investigator Group. Evaluation of platelet IIb/IIIa inhibition for prevention of ischemic complication. *JAMA* 1997;**278**(6):479–484.
33. Lincoff AM, Tcheng JE, Califf RM, *et al.* Sustained suppression of ischemic complications of coronary intervention by platelet GP IIb/IIIa blockade with abciximab: one-year outcome in the EPILOG trial. Evaluation in PTCA to improve long-term outcome with abciximab GP IIb/IIIa blockade. *Circulation* 1999;**99**(15):1951–1958.
34. Topol EJ, Moliterno DJ, Herrmann HC, *et al.* Comparison of two platelet glycoprotein IIb/IIIa inhibitors, tirofiban and abciximab, for the prevention of ischemic events with percutaneous coronary revascularization. *N Engl J Med* 2001;**344**(25):1888–1894.
35. Kastrati A, Mehilli J, Schuhlen H, *et al.* A clinical trial of abciximab in elective percutaneous coronary intervention after pretreatment with clopidogrel. *N Engl J Med* 2004;**350**(3):232–238.
36. Mehilli J, Kastrati A, Schuhlen H, *et al.* Randomized clinical trial of abciximab in diabetic patients undergoing elective percutaneous coronary interventions after treatment with a high loading dose of clopidogrel. *Circulation* 2004;**110**(24):3627–3635.
37. Lincoff AM, Bittl JA, Harrington RA, *et al.* Bivalirudin and provisional glycoprotein IIb/IIIa blockade compared with heparin and planned glycoprotein

IIb/IIIa blockade during percutaneous coronary intervention: REPLACE-2 randomized trial. *JAMA* 2003;**289**(7):853–863.

38. van den Brand M, Laarman GJ, Steg PG, *et al.* Assessment of coronary angiograms prior to and after treatment with abciximab, and the outcome of angioplasty in refractory unstable angina patients. Angiographic results from the CAPTURE trial. *Eur Heart J* 1999;**20**(21):1572–1578.
39. Hamm CW, Heeschen C, Goldmann B, *et al.* Benefit of abciximab in patients with refractory unstable angina in relation to serum troponin T levels. c7E3 Fab Antiplatelet Therapy in Unstable Refractory Angina (CAPTURE) Study Investigators. *N Engl J Med* 1999;**340**(21):1623–1629.
40. Neumann FJ, Kastrati A, Schmitt C, *et al.* Effect of glycoprotein IIb/IIIa receptor blockade with abciximab on clinical and angiographic restenosis rate after the placement of coronary stents following acute myocardial infarction. *J Am Coll Cardiol* 2000;**35**(4):915–921.
41. The ERASER Investigators. Acute platelet inhibition with abciximab does not reduce in-stent restenosis (ERASER study). *Circulation* 1999;**100**(8):799–806.
42. Simoons ML. Effect of glycoprotein IIb/IIIa receptor blocker abciximab on outcome in patients with acute coronary syndromes without early coronary revascularization: the GUSTO IV-ACS randomized trial. *Lancet* 2001;**357**(9272):1915–1924.
43. Ottervanger JP, Armstrong P, Barnathan ES, *et al.* Long-term results after the glycoprotein IIb/IIIa inhibitor abciximab in unstable angina: one-year survival in the GUSTO IV-ACS (Global Use of Strategies To Open Occluded Coronary Arteries IV — Acute Coronary Syndrome) Trial. *Circulation* 2003;**107**(3):437–442.
44. De Luca G, Suryapranata H, Stone GW, *et al.* Abciximab as adjunctive therapy to reperfusion in acute ST-segment elevation myocardial infarction: a meta-analysis of randomized trials. *JAMA* 2005;**293**(14):1759–1765.
45. Savonitto S, Armstrong PW, Lincoff AM, *et al.* Risk of intracranial hemorrhage with combined fibrinolytic and glycoprotein IIb/IIIa inhibitor therapy in acute myocardial infarction. Dichotomous response as a function of age in the GUSTO V trial. *Eur Heart J* 2003;**24**(20):1807–1814.
46. The Assessment of the Safety and Efficacy of a New Thrombolytic Regimen (ASSENT)-3 Investigators. Efficacy and safety of tenecteplase in combination with enoxaparin, abciximab, or unfractionated heparin: the ASSENT-3 randomized trial in acute myocardial infarction. *Lancet* 2001;**358**(9282):605–613.

47. Brener SJ, Barr LA, Burchenal JE, *et al.* Randomized, placebo-controlled trial of platelet glycoprotein IIb/IIIa blockade with primary angioplasty for acute myocardial infarction. ReoPro and Primary PTCA Organization and Randomized Trial (RAPPORT) Investigators. *Circulation* 1998;**98**(8): 734–741.
48. Antoniucci D, Rodriguez A, Hempel A, *et al.* A randomized trial comparing primary infarct artery stenting with or without abciximab in acute myocardial infarction. *J Am Coll Cardiol* 2003;**42**(11):1879–1885.
49. Chan AW, Chew DP, Bhatt DL, *et al.* Long-term mortality benefit with the combination of stents and abciximab for cardiogenic shock complicating acute myocardial infarction. *Am J Cardiol* 2002;**89**(2):132–136.
50. Stone GW, Grines CL, Cox DA, *et al.* Comparison of angioplasty with stenting, with or without abciximab, in acute myocardial infarction. *N Engl J Med* 2002;**346**(13):957–966.
51. Montalescot G, Barragan P, Wittenberg O, *et al.* Platelet glycoprotein IIb/IIIa inhibition with coronary stenting for acute myocardial infarction. *N Engl J Med* 2001;**344**(25):1895–1903.
52. Montalescot G, Borentain M, Payot L, *et al.* Early versus late administration of glycoprotein IIb/IIIa inhibitors in primary percutaneous coronary intervention of acute ST-segment elevation myocardial infarction: a meta-analysis. *JAMA* 2004;**292**(3):362–366.
53. Peerlinck K, De Lepeleire I, Goldberg M, *et al.* MK-383 (L-700,462), a selective nonpeptide platelet glycoprotein IIb/IIIa antagonist, is active in man. *Circulation* 1993;**88**(4 Pt 1):1512–1517.
54. The RESTORE Investigators. Effects of platelet glycoprotein IIb/IIIa blockade with tirofiban on adverse cardiac events in patients with unstable angina or acute myocardial infarction undergoing coronary angioplasty. Randomized Efficacy Study of Tirofiban for Outcomes and REstenosis. *Circulation* 1997;**96**(5):1445–1453.
55. Cannon CP, Weintraub WS, Demopoulos LA, *et al.* Comparison of early invasive and conservative strategies in patients with unstable coronary syndromes treated with the glycoprotein IIb/IIIa inhibitor tirofiban. *N Engl J Med* 2001;**344**(25):1879–1887.
56. Platelet Receptor Inhibition in Ischemic Syndrome Management (PRISM) Study Investigators. A comparison of aspirin plus tirofiban with aspirin plus heparin for unstable angina. *N Engl J Med* 1998;**338**(21):1498–1505.
57. Platelet Receptor Inhibition in Ischemic Syndrome Management in Patients Limited by Unstable Signs and Symptoms (PRISM-PLUS) Study Investigators. Inhibition of the platelet glycoprotein IIb/IIIa receptor with tirofiban

in unstable angina and non-Q-wave myocardial infarction. *N Engl J Med* 1998;**338**(21):1488–1497.

58. The PURSUIT Trial Investigators. Inhibition of platelet glycoprotein IIb/IIIa with eptifibatide in patients with acute coronary syndromes. Platelet glycoprotein IIb/IIIa in unstable angina: receptor suppression using integrilin therapy. *N Engl J Med* 1998;**339**(7):436–443.
59. The PARAGON Investigators. International, randomized, controlled trial of lamifiban (a platelet glycoprotein IIb/IIIa inhibitor), heparin, or both in unstable angina. *Circulation* 1998;**97**(24):2386–2395.
60. Platelet IIb/IIIa Antagonism for the Reduction of Acute Coronary Syndrome Events in a Global Organization Network. Randomized, placebo-controlled trial of titrated intravenous lamifiban for acute coronary syndromes. *Circulation* 2002;**105**(3):316–321.
61. Boersma E, Harrington RA, Moliterno DJ, *et al.* Platelet glycoprotein IIb/IIIa inhibitors in acute coronary syndromes. *Lancet* 2002;**360**(9329):342–343.
62. Valgimigli M, Percoco G, Barbieri D, *et al.* The additive value of tirofiban administered with the high-dose bolus in the prevention of ischemic complications during high-risk coronary angioplasty: the ADVANCE Trial. *J Am Coll Cardiol* 2004;**44**(1):14–19.
63. The IMPACT-II Investigators. Randomized placebo-controlled trial of effect of eptifibatide on complications of percutaneous coronary intervention: IMPACT-II. Integrilin to minimise platelet aggregation and coronary thrombosis-II. *Lancet* 2002;**349**(9063):1422–1428.
64. The ESPRIT Investigators. Novel dosing regimen of eptifibatide in planned coronary stent implantation (ESPRIT): a randomized, placebo-controlled trial. *Lancet* 2000;**356**(9247):2037–2044.
65. van't Hof AW, Ernst N, de Boer MJ, *et al.* Facilitation of primary coronary angioplasty by early start of a glycoprotein 2b/3a inhibitor: results of the ongoing tirofiban in myocardial infarction evaluation (On-TIME) trial. *Eur Heart J* 2004;**25**(10):837–846.
66. Cohen M, Gensini GF, Maritz F, *et al.* The safety and efficacy of subcutaneous enoxaparin versus intravenous unfractionated heparin and tirofiban versus placebo in the treatment of acute ST-segment elevation myocardial infarction patients ineligible for reperfusion (TETAMI): a randomized trial. *J Am Coll Cardiol* 2003;**42**(8):1348–1356.
67. Ault KA, Cannon CP, Mitchell J, *et al.* Platelet activation in patients after an acute coronary syndrome: results from the TIMI-12 trial. Thrombolysis in myocardial infarction. *J Am Coll Cardiol* 1999;**33**(3):634–639.

68. O'Neill WW, Serruys P, Knudtson M, *et al.* Long-term treatment with a platelet glycoprotein-receptor antagonist after percutaneous coronary revascularization. EXCITE trial investigators. evaluation of oral xemilofiban in controlling thrombotic events. *N Engl J Med* 2000;**342**(18):1316–1324.
69. Cannon CP, McCabe CH, Wilcox RG, *et al.* Oral glycoprotein IIb/IIIa inhibition with orbofiban in patients with unstable coronary syndromes (OPUS-TIMI 16) trial. *Circulation* 2000;**102**(2):149–156.
70. The SYMPHONY Investigators. Comparison of sibrafiban with aspirin for prevention of cardiovascular events after acute coronary syndromes: a randomized trial. Sibrafiban versus aspirin to yield maximum protection from ischemic heart events post-acute coronary syndromes. *Lancet* 2000;**355**(9201):337–345.
71. Second SYMPHONY Investigators. Randomized trial of aspirin, sibrafiban, or both for secondary prevention after acute coronary syndromes. *Circulation* 2001;**103**(13):1727–1733.
72. Topol EJ, Easton D, Harrington RA, *et al.* Randomized, double-blind, placebo-controlled, international trial of the oral IIb/IIIa antagonist lotrafiban in coronary and cerebrovascular disease. *Circulation* 2003;**108**(4):399–406.
73. Leebeek FW, Boersma E, Cannon CP, *et al.* Oral glycoprotein IIb/IIIa receptor inhibitors in patients with cardiovascular disease: why were the results so unfavourable. *Eur Heart J* 2002;**23**(6):444–457.
74. Adderley SR, Fitzgerald DJ. Glycoprotein IIb/IIIa antagonists induce apoptosis in rat cardiomyocytes by caspase-3 activation. *J Biol Chem* 2000;**275**(8):5760–5766.
75. Stone GW, Bertrand M, Colombo A, *et al.* Acute Catheterization and Urgent Intervention Triage strategY (ACUITY) trial: study design and rationale. *Am Heart J* 2004;**148**(5):764–775.

4 ADP Receptor Antagonists

Juhana Karha and Christopher P. Cannon

Adenosine Diphosphate Receptor

The platelet has a variety of membrane receptors that recognize nucleic acids and their metabolites as ligands. The nomenclature of the receptors includes the letter P to designate their ligands as purines. The P1 purinoceptors are activated by adenosine. The P2 receptors, bound by the adenosine nucleotides adenosine triphosphate (ATP) and adenosine diphosphate (ADP), are categorized into three types: $P2X_1$, $P2Y_1$, and $P2Y_{12}$. The $P2X_1$ receptor is a platelet membrane ion channel allowing rapid calcium ion influx upon activation by ATP (Fig. 1). The subsequent increase in intracellular calcium concentration leads to platelet shape change and platelet aggregation. To date the $P2X_1$ receptor has not been utilized as a clinical target in cardiovascular pharmacology, but it certainly represents an untapped possibility for future investigation and drug development.

The P2Y receptors ($P2Y_1$ and $P2Y_{12}$) are transmembrane proteins with seven hydrophobic domains (Fig. 1). The receptors are bound and activated on the outer surface by ADP. The number of binding sites on the platelet outer surface is fairly small, estimated at less than 1000 per cell. The $P2Y_1$ receptor is coupled to a G-protein, which mediates a cascade leading to mobilization of intracellular calcium stores. The resulting increase in intracellular calcium concentration then leads to a change in the shape of the platelet, followed by aggregation of platelets and the formation of the platelet plug. The $P2Y_1$ receptor is an attractive target for drug development. Supporting this notion are the findings from animal studies where in mice the deficiency of this receptor causes less thrombosis (in response to a broad

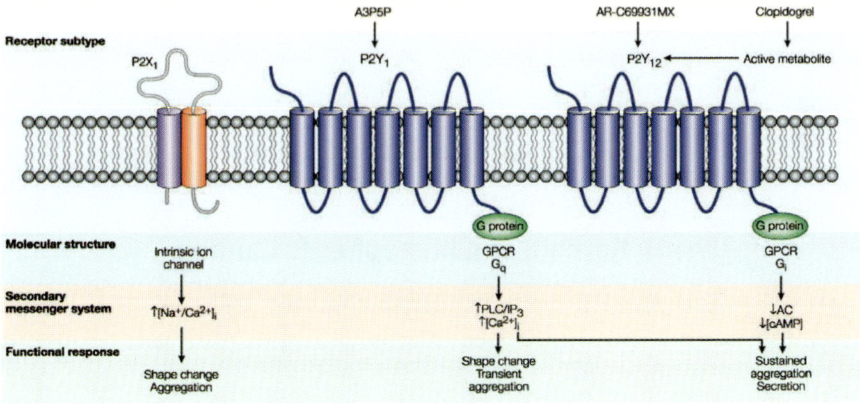

Fig. 1. The three different subtypes of ADP receptors: $P2X_1$, $P2Y_1$, and $P2Y_{12}$ (reprinted with permission from the Nature Publishing Group).

range of agonists such as ADP, collagen, and epinephrine) and increased bleeding time, but no increase in the amount of spontaneous bleeding.

The $P2Y_{12}$ receptor is among the most studied and utilized in pharmacotherapy of cardiovascular disease. It is activated by ADP and coupled to a G-protein. In this case, the effect of the receptor activation is inhibition of intracellular adenylyl cyclase. The resultant biochemical cascade ultimately amplifies the process of platelet activation and aggregation thus sustaining ongoing thrombus formation. Recently, an important milestone in platelet physiology was reached when this receptor was cloned by Hollopeter and coworkers[1] Underscoring the importance of the platelet $P2Y_{12}$ receptor is that it serves as the target for the two thienopyridines, clopidogrel and ticlopidine, in current clinical use.

Ticlopidine

As the first ADP receptor antagonist approved for clinical use, ticlopidine was a significant addition to physicians' armamentarium. The introduction of ticlopidine represented the first new medication targeting the platelet in decades. Previously, the platelet cyclo-oxygenases and phosphodiesterases were the major targets of pharmacotherapy with aspirin and dipyridamole, respectively. Ticlopidine was introduced under the trade name Ticlid™ in the United States.

Ticlopidine, the first in the class of thienopyridine medications, blocks the ADP receptor and thus provides inhibition of a pivotal pathway in the physiology of platelets. The biochemical structure is *5-[(2-chlorophenyl)methyl]-4,5,6,7-tetrahydrothieno [3,2-c] pyridine hydrochloride*. Its biochemical structure is depicted in Fig. 2. It is a prodrug that is converted into the bioactive compound by a liver cytochrome P450 3A4 enzyme. This active metabolite irreversibly binds the platelet membrane ADP $P2Y_{12}$receptor, forming a disulfide bond and permanently inactivating the receptor. This inactivation interferes in a dose-dependent manner with the process of platelet aggregation.

Ticlopidine is dosed at 250 mg twice daily. Antacid medications interfere with ticlopidine absorption and reduce it according to some estimates by 18%. Conversely, ticlopidine absorption may be augmented by concomitant intake of foods that contain high amounts of fat. Peak plasma concentration of ticlopidine occurs one to three hours after the administration of a single oral dose of 250 mg, as up to 90% of the medication is absorbed. A large

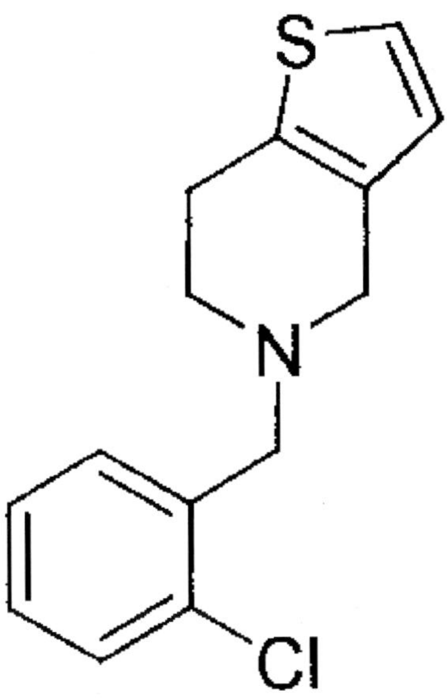

Fig. 2. The molecular structure of ticlopidine.

percentage of ticlopidine (> 98%) is bound to albumin and other plasma proteins, and on twice-a-day dosing the drug accumulates over two to three weeks. Up to 13 different metabolites of ticlopidine have been identified. After steady state has been reached, the elimination half-life of ticlopidine is up to 96 hours. Similarly, the elimination half-life after only a single dose is 24 to 36 hours. One very important feature of cardiovascular medications is speed of action, as many cardiovascular illnesses are dynamic processes that require urgent therapy. In the case of ticlopidine, a loading dose has not been well studied, and initiating therapy merely with the maintenance dosing does not result in as quick an action as is often needed in cardiovascular medicine. So in other words, ticlopidine is not suitable when rapid antiplatelet effect is desired, and this is one reason that clopidogrel has become the preferred thienopyridine medication.

Cerebrovascular disease

Multiple clinical studies have evaluated the safety and efficacy of ticlopidine in various patient populations. One of the first illnesses to be examined was cerebrovascular disease. In the Ticlopidine Aspirin Stroke Study (TASS) trial, Hass and coworkers compared ticlopidine with aspirin, the established antiplatelet treatment of choice in cerebrovascular disease. They conducted a study of 3069 patients with a recent small stroke or transient cerebral ischemia, and demonstrated that ticlopidine was superior to aspirin in reducing the incidence of stroke after three years of follow-up.[2] The risk of stroke among the patients who received ticlopidine was 10%, a significantly lower number than the 13% incidence among the control group ($p = 0.02$). Likewise, the combined risk of death or stroke was also lower in the treatment group (17% versus 19%, $p = 0.05$).

Another major endeavor in establishing ticlopidine's role in the treatment of ischemic cerebrovascular disease was the Canadian American Ticlopidine Study (CATS).[3] The CATS investigators evaluated 1072 patients with a history of a presumably thromboembolic stroke. They were randomized to receive ticlopidine versus placebo and the follow-up period extended over two years. The study demonstrated that ticlopidine reduced the combined endpoint of vascular death, stroke, or myocardial infarction compared to placebo. The incidence of the primary endpoint among patients receiving ticlopidine and placebo was 11.3% versus 14.0%, respectively, $p = 0.02$. This corresponds to a relative risk reduction with ticlopidine therapy of 23%.

The African American Antiplatelet Stroke Prevention Study randomized 1809 black men and women with a recent non-cardioembolic ischemic stroke to ticlopidine versus aspirin and followed them for two years.[4] The incidence of the primary combined endpoint of vascular death, myocardial infarction, or recurrent stroke was similar in the ticlopidine and aspirin groups: 14.7% versus 12.3%, respectively (hazard ratio with ticlopidine use 1.22, 95% confidence interval 0.94–1.57, $p = 0.12$).

Thus, in total these studies show that ticlopidine is effective in reducing adverse ischemic outcomes in patients with a prior cerebrovascular event when compared to placebo. Furthermore, there may be a modest benefit when ticlopidine is compared to aspirin in high risk populations. These investigations suggested the use of ticlopidine for the treatment of cerebral ischemia in cases of aspirin failure or when aspirin cannot be tolerated or is contraindicated.

Acute coronary syndromes

Ticlopidine has also been evaluated in patients with coronary artery disease. Addition of ticlopidine to conventional therapy without aspirin in 652 patients with unstable angina resulted in a lower rate of vascular death or myocardial infarction compared to the control group. In this study, the relative risk of the primary endpoint with ticlopidine therapy was 0.54 ($p = 0.009$) after six months of follow-up.[5]

Percutaneous coronary intervention

Another major arena of thienopyridine use has been among patients undergoing percutaneous coronary intervention with stent implantation. Hall and coworkers randomized 226 patients undergoing intravascular ultrasound guided intracoronary stent placement to a regimen of aspirin plus ticlopidine versus aspirin alone.[6] Although the study was underpowered, there was an impressive numerical difference favoring ticlopidine group in the incidence of stent thrombosis within one month of stent placement (0.8% versus 2.9%, $p = 0.2$). The Intracoronary Stenting and Antithrombotic Regimen (ISAR) was a larger study of 517 patients undergoing coronary angioplasty with stent placement.[7] The patients were randomized to receive ticlopidine plus aspirin versus oral anticoagulation with phenprocoumon plus aspirin. The 30-day incidence of the combined endpoint of cardiac death, myocardial infarction, or need for a revascularization procedure was lower in the ticlopidine group compared to the anticoagulation group (1.6% versus 6.2%, $p = 0.01$).

Another study examining the optimal antiplatelet regimen following PCI with stenting was the Multicentre Aspirin and Ticlopidine Trial after Intracoronary Stenting (MATTIS) study.[8] A total of 350 patients were randomized to treatment with ticlopidine versus oral anticoagulation following PCI with stenting. All patients received aspirin. The 30-day incidence of the combined endpoint of cardiovascular death, myocardial infarction, or repeat revascularization was lower (failing to reach statistical significance) in the ticlopidine group compared to the anticoagulation group (5.6% versus 11.0%, $p = 0.07$). In the Stent Anticoagulation Restenosis Study (STARS) by Leon *et al.* in 1653 patients undergoing coronary angioplasty with stenting, ticlopidine plus aspirin was compared in a three-arm design to antiplatelet therapy with aspirin alone as well as to a strategy of aspirin plus anticoagulation with warfarin.[9] The primary endpoint aimed at capturing the process of stent thrombosis and was defined as a 30-day composite of death, myocardial infarction, the presence of thrombus on a subsequent angiogram, or need for revascularization of the target lesion. The primary endpoint occurred in 0.5%, 3.6%, and 2.7% of the patients in the aspirin plus ticlopidine, aspirin only, and aspirin plus warfarin groups, respectively (three-way p-value = 0.001).

Bertrand and coworkers studied ticlopidine after stent implantation in the Full Anticoagulation versus Aspirin and Ticlopidine (FANTASTIC) trial.[10] A total of 485 patients undergoing elective or bailout stenting were randomized to ticlopidine versus anticoagulation with warfarin. All patients were treated with aspirin. The ticlopidine group had a lower rate of subacute (beyond the first 24 hours after PCI) stent occlusion with all events occurring within one week after PCI (0.4% versus 3.5%, $p = 0.01$). Interestingly, the rate of early thrombosis (within 24 hours of PCI) was higher in the antiplatelet therapy group compared to the anticoagulation group: 2.4% versus 0.4%, respectively, $p = 0.06$. This important observation likely reflects the delayed onset of action of ticlopidine, highlighting the need to achieve rapid therapeutic thienopyridine levels in patients who undergo coronary stent placement.

In total, these studies suggest that the addition of ticlopidine to aspirin following coronary angioplasty with stent placement reduces the risk of stent thrombosis. They also establish that antiplatelet therapy with aspirin and a thienopyridine is superior to a strategy of aspirin plus oral anticoagulation in suppressing the worrisome complication of stent thrombosis, in addition to a lower rate of major bleeding. These data along with evaluations of clopidogrel (see below) are the foundation for the universal acceptance of thienopyridine therapy for patients undergoing coronary angioplasty with stent implantation.

Coronary artery bypass graft surgery

Interestingly, highlighting the role of platelets in the pathophysiology of arterial thrombosis, ticlopidine has also been shown to reduce the rate of acute occlusion of aortocoronary venous bypass grafts compared with placebo.[11,12]

Peripheral arterial disease

Another population that appears to derive benefit from ticlopidine therapy is patients with peripheral arterial disease. The Swedish Ticlopidine Multicentre Study (STIMS) randomized 687 patients with intermittent claudication to ticlopidine 250 mg twice daily versus placebo.[13] The incidence of myocardial infarction, stroke, and transient ischemic attack (TIA) was 34% lower among patients receiving ticlopidine compared to the control group (25.7% versus 29.0%, respectively, $p < 0.05$). Likewise, the incidence of the need for vascular surgery was lower in the treatment group.[14] Other studies have demonstrated similar benefits with ticlopidine therapy in reducing vascular complications and increasing walking distance in patients with peripheral arterial disease.[13,15–17] Given the reduction in adverse cardiovascular events that ticlopidine appears to have in a broad range of cardiovascular disease, it is not surprising that an analysis of the Antiplatelet Trialists' Collaboration study, a heterogeneous population of patients at high risk for the complications of cardiovascular disease, demonstrated that use of ticlopidine was associated with a 10% lower risk of vascular events compared to use of aspirin.[18]

Despite its efficacy in suppressing adverse cardiovascular events across a wide range of vascular disease, ticlopidine is used only rarely today due to its safety with respect to hematologic aberrations. Aplastic anemia, neutropenia, thrombocytopenia, and thrombotic thrombocytopenic purpura (TTP) are possible complications of ticlopidine therapy (see below for further discussion).[19,20] Other side effects of ticlopidine include diarrhea, gastrointestinal intolerance, rash, and bleeding complications. The use of ticlopidine in pregnancy is designated with the safety category "B", that is, its use has no evidence of risk in humans.

As mentioned above, the major shortfall of ticlopidine turned out to be the idiosyncratic and severe hematologic illnesses that are associated with its clinical use. In approximately 2% of patients ticlopidine causes severe neutropenia. The incidence of neutropenia to absolute neutrophil counts (ANC) of $< 450 \times 10^6$/liter ($= 450/\text{mm}^3$) is 0.8%. About 2.4% of patients experience a fall in their ANC to below 1200×10^6/liter ($= 1200/\text{mm}^3$).

The incidence of thrombotic thrombocytopenic purpura (TTP) among patients treated with ticlopidine following coronary stent placement is 0.02% (representing a 50-fold increase compared to the incidence in general population of 0.0004%). This increase in risk of TTP is particularly significant considering the high mortality rate of over 20% associated with this disorder. TTP is a clinical entity with the presenting pentad of microangiopathic hemolytic anemia, thrombocytopenia, fever, altered mental status, and worsened renal function. TTP is caused by an acquired deficiency of plasma metalloprotease ADAMTS13, which cleaves von Willebrand's factor (vWF). The peak incidence of TTP associated with ticlopidine therapy occurs between three to four weeks after the onset of therapy, whereas peak neutropenia and aplastic anemia incidences fall on weeks 4–6 and 4–8, respectively. However, a few cases have been reported after three months of therapy.

In clinical practice, these hematologic concerns necessitated routine monitoring of leukocyte count, and careful clinical evaluation of patients who are on ticlopidine therapy. The recommendation is to routinely obtain a complete blood count with a differential count every two weeks starting in the second week of therapy. The routine monitoring can be stopped after three months of therapy. The monitoring should be intensified and extended for patients who have significant decline in their counts. Therefore, one of the by-products of this careful monitoring is an expense as a result of laboratory costs and clinic and emergency department visits. Ticlopidine should be discontinued if the absolute neutrophil count falls below 1200/mm^3. Likewise, continued monitoring and discontinuation of ticlopidine therapy are warranted if thrombocytopenia with platelet count of less than 80,000/mm^3 develops.

Ticlopidine may increase the blood levels and the biological effects of the following medications by virtue of its inhibition of the liver cytochrome P450 2C19 isoenzyme: citalopram, diazepam, methosuximide, phenytoin, propranolol, and sertraline. The cost of one-month supply (60 tablets) of ticlopidine (the generic formulation) is US$85.99 (data from drugstore.com, accessed 7/14/2005).

Clopidogrel — General Considerations

Building upon the clinical efficacy of ticlopidine, but with a more benign side effect profile, were the main challenges in the development of clopidogrel, the second drug in the thienopyridine class. Clopidogrel differs from ticlopidine by having an additional carboxymethyl group (Fig. 3). Highlighting their similar chemical structure, many of clopidogrel's functional properties are either identical or similar to those of ticlopidine. Clopidogrel

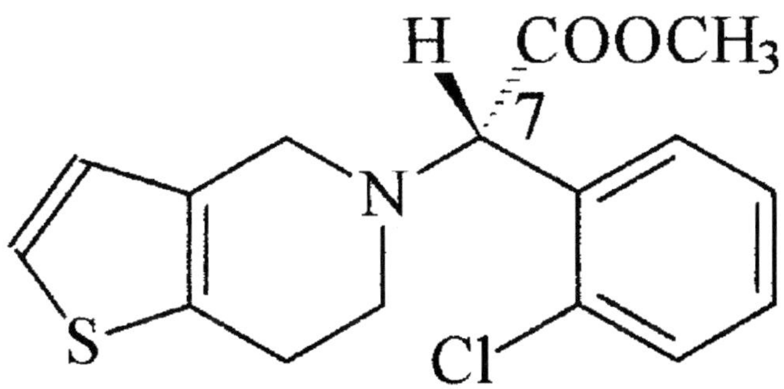

Fig. 3. The molecular structure of clopidogrel.

is inactive *in vitro* and requires metabolic activation by a liver cytochrome P450 3A4 enzyme. The active metabolite irreversibly binds the platelet membrane $P2Y_{12}$ ADP receptor and renders it permanently inactive. Biochemically this is accomplished by the drug forming a deactivating disulfide bond with the receptor. The end result of this receptor inactivation is dose-dependent inhibition of platelet aggregation.

Clopidogrel bisulfate has the chemical formula of $C_{16}H_{16}ClNO_2S \bullet H_2SO_4$, with a molecular weight of 419.9 $g mol^{-1}$ and its chemical structure is designated as *methyl(+)-(S)-alpha-(2-chlorophenyl)-6,7-dihydrothieno[3,2-c] pyridine-5(4H)-acetate sulfate*. Orally administered clopidogrel is a white powder, which is insoluble in water at neutral pH, but at $pH = 1$ it is freely soluble. The specific optical rotation of the molecule is $+56°$. The plasma concentration of the parent compound is very low, and the main (also biologically inactive) circulating metabolite is a carboxylic acid derivative. Following ^{14}C-labeled clopidogrel, 50% is excreted in urine and 46% in feces during the five days after dosing. The elimination half-life of the main circulating metabolite is eight hours (after both single and repeat dosing), and it is not altered by concomitant food intake. No dosage adjustment is needed for women, the elderly or patients with impaired renal function. However, pharmacokinetic differences due to race have not been studied.

The Food and Drug Administration (FDA) approved clopidogrel (trade name Plavix™) for clinical use for the prevention of thrombotic complications of atherosclerotic disease in November 1997. The approved daily dose was 75 mg. Initial investigations evaluating clopidogrel had selected this particular dose because it produced inhibition of platelet aggregation equivalent to that achieved with the clinically used dose of 250 mg of ticlopidine twice daily. Daily clopidogrel at the 75 mg dose requires three to seven days to reach maximal antiplatelet effect. With the 75 mg dose, the maximal level of platelet aggregation inhibition is 40%–60%, as measured by optical aggregometry (utilizing 10 μM ADP as the agonist). However, a significant amount of inter-individual variability exists in the amount of clopidogrel's antiplatelet effect. Upon cessation of therapy (once a steady state level has been reached), platelet function returns to normal after about five days.

As is the case with other antiplatelet agents, the major side effect of clopidogrel is bleeding. This is especially important as many of the indications for clopidogrel therapy also call for treatment with aspirin. In addition, some of the patients who derive benefit with respect to ischemic endpoints from dual antiplatelet therapy, also have illnesses that are best managed with oral anticoagulation with warfarin. In these cases of "triple therapy," cardiologists have to weigh carefully the incremental benefit afforded by the addition of clopidogrel against the increased bleeding risk.[21] Other possible and relatively common side effects include gastrointestinal distress, rash (4%), and abnormalities in liver function tests (leading to discontinuation in 0.11%). The severe complication of thrombotic thrombocytopenic purpura (TTP) is much less common with clopidogrel therapy than it is with the other thienopyridine, ticlopidine. It occurs in less than about four cases per million (according to post-marketing data contained in the package insert of Plavix™) of the patients and has been reported in the first two weeks of therapy. The use of clopidogrel in pregnancy is designated with the safety category "B", i.e. its use has no evidence of risk in humans.

As clopidogrel is converted into the active metabolite by the liver cytochrome P450 3A4 enzyme (CYP3A4), drug-drug interactions may exist. The macrolide antibiotics, clarithromycin and erythromycin, inhibit CYP3A4 and might theoretically attenuate clopidogrel action. On the contrary, rifampin and the over-the-counter herbal supplement St. John's wort induce CYP3A4 and may thus potentiate the effects of clopidogrel. Reported concerns about the interaction between atorvastatin and clopidogrel (CYP3A4 competitive inhibition leading to a smaller quantity of the active metabolite of clopidogrel) have been inconsistent.[22–24] Currently, no clinical interaction has been seen.

In addition to inhibiting platelet aggregation, clopidogrel also exerts actions that suppress the pro-inflammatory effects that platelets mediate. Clopidogrel, via down-stream effects following the binding of the $P2Y_{12}$ receptor, reduces the expression of P-selectin and CD40 ligand, and thus reduces platelet-neutrophil and platelet-monocyte aggregates. Quinn and colleagues demonstrated that clopidogrel pre-treatment before a percutaneous coronary intervention was associated with less platelet expression of P-selectin and CD40 ligand.[25] Vivekananthan *et al.* showed that clopidogrel pre-treatment may attenuate the peri-PCI increase in high sensitivity C-reactive protein by 65%.[26] However, preliminary data from the

CURE trial found no reduction in C-reactive protein between clopidogrel and placebo groups.[27]

At times, the cost of Plavix™ is a significant consideration as physicians evaluate the advantages and disadvantages of clopidogrel therapy for an individual patient. According to a recent pricing, the supply of Plavix™ (75 mg daily) for 30 days costs US$114.99 (data from drugstore.com, accessed on 7/14/2005). However, clopidogrel therapy has been shown to be cost-effective following both PCI and ACS.[28,29]

Clopidogrel in Atherothrombotic Disease

The trial that launched clopidogrel as a major drug in the pharmacotherapy of vascular disease was the Clopidogrel versus Aspirin in Patients at Risk of Ischemic Events (CAPRIE) trial.[30] It was a very large trial with 19,185 patients randomized to antiplatelet therapy. The study population was a heterogeneous group of patients with vascular disease. The inclusion criteria focused on three different presentations. Patients were required to meet one of the following criteria: ischemic stroke in the past six months, myocardial infarction in the prior 35 days, or intermittent claudication. Ultimately these subgroups consisted of 6431, 6302, and 6452 patients, respectively. Given the size of the overall trial, even these subgroups were large in size. The patients were randomized to receive clopidogrel 75 mg daily versus aspirin 325 mg daily for a mean duration of 1.9 years. Matching placebos were used in place of both aspirin and clopidogrel, and the study was double blinded. The patients underwent periodic monitoring of the leukocyte and platelet counts to protect against the possible occurrence of leukopenia or thrombocytopenia.

The primary endpoint in the CAPRIE trial was a composite of vascular death, myocardial infarction, and ischemic stroke. The annual event rate of the primary endpoint was lower among patients who received clopidogrel than those who were treated with aspirin: 5.3% versus 5.8%, respectively, $p = 0.043$. This corresponds to a relative risk reduction with clopidogrel therapy of 8.7% (95% CI: 0.3%–16.5%). Most of this difference was a result of a lower rate of myocardial infarction among the clopidogrel-treated patients (absolute number of myocardial infarctions in the two groups: $n = 275$ versus $n = 333$, for clopidogrel and aspirin groups, respectively).

All-cause annual mortality was similar in the two groups: 3.05% and 3.11% in the clopidogrel and aspirin groups, respectively, $p = 0.71$. A retrospective study of the CAPRIE trial showed that randomization to clopidogrel was associated with a 19.2% relative risk reduction ($p = 0.008$) in the risk of sustaining a fatal or non-fatal acute myocardial infarction.[31] This benefit was noted across all patient risk profiles, that is to say, patients at low risk of developing myocardial infarction received similar benefit from clopidogrel therapy compared to patients at high risk.

In a further analysis of the CAPRIE study, the following clinical variables were associated with greater absolute risk reduction observed with clopidogrel therapy: history of coronary artery bypass graft operation (15.9% versus 22.3%; relative risk reduction, RRR 28.9%),[32] history of multiple ischemic events (18.4% versus 20.4%, RRR 10.0%),[33] clinical involvement of multiple vascular beds (17.4% versus 19.8%, RRR 12.4%), diabetes mellitus (15.6% versus 17.7%, RRR 12.5%, and insulin treated diabetes (17.7% versus 21.5%, RRR 16.7%).[34] Rehospitalization for ischemic or bleeding events was also reduced with clopidogrel therapy compared with aspirin.[35] Interestingly, the CAPRIE Actual Practice Rates Analysis (CAPRA) study suggested that the risk of adverse vascular events is higher in the "real-world" practice compared to clinical trials, such as CAPRIE.[36] Accordingly, the benefit of a therapy such as clopidogrel would tend to be greater in clinical practice than that seen in a clinical trial setting.

Regarding safety endpoints in the CAPRIE trial, clopidogrel was well tolerated. Rash (6%) and diarrhea (4%) were more common among the clopidogrel-treated patients than among those who received aspirin (5% and 3%, respectively). Clopidogrel therapy, notably, was associated with a lower incidence of bleeding complications compared to aspirin (9.3% versus 9.3%, respectively; for gastrointestinal bleeding: 2.0% versus 2.7%, respectively). The rate of intracranial hemorrhage was similar with clopidogrel compared to aspirin (0.35% versus 0.49%, respectively). The rates of neutropenia and severe neutropenia were similar among patients treated with clopidogrel and aspirin. Neutropenia occurred in 0.10% and 0.17% of the patients in the clopidogrel and aspirin groups, respectively, and the corresponding rates of severe neutropenia were 0.05% and 0.04%, respectively. No increase in plasma cholesterol level was noted in the clopidogrel group. Thus, in total, the CAPRIE trial demonstrated that clopidogrel 75 mg daily is an effective and safe secondary prevention treatment among patients with vascular disease. Much of the benefit seen in the trial was due to a lower rate of myocardial infarction.

Clopidogrel in Cerebrovascular Disease

No placebo controlled outcome trials exist for clopidogrel and aspirin. The benefit of thienopyridine in cerebrovascular disease is largely based on ticlopidine. One trial evaluated the role of adding aspirin to clopidogrel. The Management of Atherothrombosis with Clopidogrel in High Risk Patients with Recent TIA or Ischemic Stroke (MATCH) trial compared clopidogrel 75 mg daily plus aspirin 75 mg daily to clopidogrel alone in 7599 patients with a recent stroke or TIA and thus was a study of aspirin on a background of clopidogrel.[37] Follow-up was for 18 months. The incidence of the primary combined endpoint of vascular death, myocardial infarction, ischemic stroke, or rehospitalization for acute ischemia in any vascular bed was similar in the two groups: 15.7% versus 16.7% for dual therapy versus clopidogrel only groups, respectively, $p = 0.24$. However, dual antiplatelet therapy was associated with an increased risk of a life-threatening bleed (2.6% versus 1.3%, $p < 0.001$). Considering the MATCH trial, it appears that in this population clopidogrel alone is superior to the combination of clopidogrel plus aspirin with similar efficacy, but less bleeding.

A recent Clopidogrel and Aspirin for Reduction of Emboli in Symptomatic Carotid Stenosis (CARESS) trial randomized 107 patients with a symptomatic carotid stenosis and transcranial Doppler evidence of microembolization to receive clopidogrel versus placebo for seven days. All patients received aspirin throughout the study period. A repeat examination performed on day 7 revealed that patients in the aspirin plus clopidogrel group had fewer microemboli compared to patients in the aspirin monotherapy group (44% versus 73%, $p = 0.005$). This study provides further supportive evidence for the use of dual antiplatelet therapy in cerebrovascular disease compared with aspirin.[38]

There are several other trials in progress that will also provide further insight into the combination of aspirin plus clopidogrel versus aspirin in the management of cerebrovascular disease, Antithrombotic Therapy in Acute Recovered cerebral Ischaemia (ATARI) trial, Aortic arch-Related Cerebral

Hazard (ARCH) trial, Secondary Prevention of Small Subcortical Strokes (SPS3) trial, and the Fast Assessment of Stroke and Transient ischemic attack to prevent Early Recurrence (FASTER) trial.[39] All of these trials compare aspirin plus clopidogrel to aspirin, except for the ARCH trial in which the comparator groups are combination of aspirin plus clopidogrel versus a strategy of oral anticoagulation.

Multiple ongoing trials are further delineating the optimal antiplatelet regimen in the treatment of cerebrovascular disease. The Prevention Regimen For Effectively avoiding Second Strokes (PRoFESS) trial is a 15,500-patient study investigating therapies for prevention of second stroke. Patients with a recent ischemic stroke (within 90 days) will be enrolled with an anticipated follow-up duration of four years. The two-by-two factorial design compares on the one hand clopidogrel versus extended-release dipyridamole plus aspirin. The other comparison will be between telmisartan and placebo (with blood pressure control achieved with other agents). The primary endpoint will be time to second stroke.

In choosing a long-term antiplatelet regimen for patients after they have had a stroke or a transient ischemic attack, preferable options at present are either clopidogrel or a combination of aspirin plus extended-release dipyridamole (Aggrenox™). However, aspirin monotherapy continues to be another acceptable alternative.[40]

Clopidogrel in Cardiovascular Disease

Clopidogrel is a widely used medication in the management of cardiovascular disease. It is used in the treatment of acute ischemic coronary syndromes, in secondary prevention of ischemic heart disease, as an adjunctive therapy for coronary angioplasty procedures, and following coronary stent implantation. A number of clinical trials have established clopidogrel as an important agent in the treatment of cardiovascular disease.

Percutaneous coronary intervention

The Clopidogrel Aspirin Stent International Cooperative Study (CLASSICS) was the first major study to evaluate the use of clopidogrel in the setting of a percutaneous coronary intervention (PCI).[41] A total of 1020 patients undergoing PCI with stenting were randomized to receive clopidogrel or ticlopidine after the PCI. All patients received aspirin 325 mg daily. In addition, all patients received a thienopyridine agent: either ticlopidine 250 mg twice daily, clopidogrel 75 mg daily, or clopidogrel with a loading dose of 300 mg, followed by clopidogrel 75 mg daily. The three groups experienced similar efficacy of antiplatelet therapy, but clopidogrel was safer and better tolerated than ticlopidine.

In addition to the CLASSICS trial, clopidogrel has been compared to ticlopidine in multiple interventional cardiology studies. Bhatt and colleagues performed a meta-analysis of these comparisons (both randomized trials and observational studies) and demonstrated that patients treated with clopidogrel were less likely to experience a major adverse cardiac event (MACE) in the 30 days following PCI compared to those treated with ticlopidine. The absolute MACE rates were 2.1% and 4.0% for clopidogrel and ticlopidine, respectively, and the odds ratio for an ischemic event was 0.72, $p = 0.002$, in favor of clopidogrel.[42] Mortality was also lower in the clopidogrel group: 0.48% versus 1.09%, $p = 0.003$.

Unstable angina/non-ST-elevation myocardial infarction

The first major trial investigating clopidogrel among patients with an acute presentation of coronary artery disease was the Clopidogrel in Unstable angina to prevent Recurrent Events (CURE) trial.[43] The CURE trial randomized 12,562 patients with unstable angina or non-ST-elevation myocardial infarction (NSTEMI) to receive aspirin plus clopidogrel versus aspirin plus placebo. The treatment group received a loading dose of clopidogrel 300 mg, followed by a daily dose of 75 mg for three to 12 months (mean nine months) duration. Aspirin dose was 75–325 mg daily. The patients in the clopidogrel group had a lower incidence of the primary combined endpoint of cardiovascular death, myocardial infarction, or stroke compared to the patients in the aspirin monotherapy arm (9.3% versus 11.4%, relative risk with clopidogrel as compared with placebo 0.80, 95% confidence interval 0.72 to 0.90, $p < 0.001$). The beneficial effect of clopidogrel emerged within 24 hours of randomization, and treated patients had a highly significant risk reduction of 21% at 30 days ($p < 0.001$). Patients derived further benefit during the remainder of the study period, demonstrating that clopidogrel continues to add benefit beyond the first 30 days. Subgroup analyses demonstrated that clopidogrel benefit existed regardless of concomitant other medications such as angiotensin-converting enzyme inhibitors, beta-adrenergic blockers, lipid-lowering agents, or heparin. Furthermore, it did not matter whether patients underwent a revascularization procedure after randomization or not. Bleeding complications were significantly increased in the dual antiplatelet therapy arm as the incidence of major bleeding was 3.7% versus 2.7% in the aspirin only group, $p = 0.001$. However, there was a nonsignificant increase in the incidence of life-threatening bleeding in the clopidogrel group: 2.1% versus 1.8%, $p = 0.13$. The dose of aspirin influenced the bleeding rate with low dose aspirin (75–100 mg daily) having about 40% lower rate than seen with higher aspirin doses (200–325 mg daily). Among patients receiving clopidogrel, the rates of major bleeding for 75–100 mg and 200–325 mg doses of aspirin were 3.0% and 4.9%, respectively.[44] These data suggest that low dose aspirin has a favorable safety profile.

Of note, only 6% of the patients in the clopidogrel arm of the CURE trial were treated aggressively with an early invasive strategy and glycoprotein IIb/IIIa inhibition. Patients who derived greater relative risk reduction with clopidogrel therapy (i.e. benefited more from clopidogrel) were those with a history of a prior revascularization procedure.[45] A retrospective analysis of the CURE study demonstrated that the benefit of clopidogrel (versus placebo) was similar in patients at low, intermediate, and high risk.[46] Patients were divided into three risk groups according to their TIMI risk score (0–2, 3–4, and 5–7) and the endpoint was a composite of cardiovascular death, myocardial infarction, and stroke. The relative risk reduction with clopidogrel therapy among the patients with low, intermediate, and high risk was 0.29, 0.15, and 0.27, respectively.

The PCI-CURE substudy was a pre-specified subgroup analysis of the patients in the CURE trial who went on to undergo PCI.[47] In this substudy of 2658 patients, the mean duration of treatment (clopidogrel versus placebo) prior to the angioplasty procedure was ten days. The relative risk of the primary combined endpoint (cardiovascular death, myocardial infarction, or the need for an urgent revascularization procedure) at 30 days among the patients treated with clopidogrel was 0.70 (0.50–0.97, $p = 0.03$), corresponding to a greater relative risk reduction than what was noted in the overall trial. The benefit was seen as early as two days after PCI and all subgroups seemed to benefit. Once again highlighting the importance of continued therapy, the patients in the clopidogrel arm continued to derive further clinical risk reduction from 31 days (after the PCI) to end of follow-up. The incidence of the primary endpoint of cardiovascular death or myocardial infarction at the PCI-CURE substudy end was 8.8% versus 12.6% for clopidogrel and placebo groups, respectively ($p = 0.002$). This represents a large absolute reduction in events with approximately four events prevented per 100 patients treated for one year (versus one month). No increase was noted in the risk of major bleeding in the PCI-CURE substudy.

The CURE study supports the treatment of patients with non-ST elevation acute coronary syndromes with aspirin and clopidogrel. Following the review of the CURE trial findings, in February of 2002, the Food and Drug Administration (FDA) approved the clopidogrel 300 mg loading dose followed by 75 mg daily for treatment of acute coronary syndromes.

The two prevailing strategies for initiating clopidogrel therapy for a patient with an acute coronary syndrome (ACS) are (1) immediate start of clopidogrel with a loading dose (300–600 mg) and (2) delay until after coronary angiography, and then either start of clopidogrel as PCI is undertaken or continued withholding of clopidogrel as the patient waits to undergo CABG surgery. The two strategies differ in that immediate clopidogrel therapy affords the benefits of reducing early ischemic events and of pretreatment prior to PCI. On the other hand, it is associated with greater bleeding should the patient require early CABG surgery (within five days). The initiation of clopidogrel therapy yields an approximate 1% absolute reduction in ischemic events within the first 24 hours.[48] In addition, for those patients who go onto PCI, there is a 30% relative reduction in the incidence of cardiovascular death or MI associated with the pretreatment.[47] Interestingly, patients who ultimately require early CABG are actually at particularly high risk of ischemic events and derive most of clopidogrel's benefit in the period between their presentation with ACS and the CABG surgery.[49] In all, these CABG patients have a 3.5% absolute reduction in the combined endpoint of cardiovascular death, MI, or stroke compared to patients who are treated in the pre-CABG period with aspirin only.[49] This is roughly equivalent to the 3.3% excess bleeding (consisting of moderate bleeding, with no increase in severe or life-threatening bleeding) with clopidogrel seen in the CURE study.[49] So, even for those ACS patients who require CABG (currently about 11% of the patients in the CRUSADE registry), the benefits are comparable to the risks. Thus, the evidence does not support the strategy of withholding the effective therapy of immediate clopidogrel loading from a great majority of patients, for the purpose of trading less moderate bleeding for more ischemic cardiovascular adverse events in a minority of patients.

The Clopidogrel for the Reduction of Events During Observation (CREDO) examined the role of early and sustained clopidogrel therapy in percutaneous coronary intervention.[50] It sought to test the dual hypotheses that clinical outcomes following percutaneous coronary intervention would be improved with clopidogrel therapy that (1) was initiated before the procedure and that (2) lasted for an extended duration following the procedure. A total of 2116 patients undergoing elective PCI (or considered at high likelihood of requiring a PCI) were randomized to a clopidogrel loading dose (300 mg) versus placebo to be administered three to 24 hours (mean 9.8 hours) before the PCI. All patients received aspirin therapy throughout the study and clopidogrel treatment (75 mg) for the first 28 days after the PCI. Intravenous platelet glycoprotein IIb/IIIa inhibitor use was allowed in the trial per operator preference. The primary endpoint in the analysis that examined the loading of clopidogrel prior to the PCI was a 28-day incidence of the composite of death, myocardial infarction, or urgent target vessel revascularization.

Clopidogrel pretreatment was associated with a similar rate of primary endpoint compared to the no-pretreatment arm of the study (6.8% versus 8.3%, $p = 0.23$). However, if only those patients who had received their clopidogrel loading dose at least six hours prior to the angioplasty procedure were considered (that is six to 24 hours before PCI), then clopidogrel loading did seem to have a benefit (5.8% versus 9.4%, $p = 0.051$). The incidence of major bleeding through one year was numerically higher among the long-term clopidogrel group compared to the aspirin only group (8.8% versus 6.7%, respectively), but failed to reach statistical significance ($p = 0.07$).

The second hypothesis was then evaluated by administering the patients in the treatment group long-term clopidogrel (75 mg daily) through 12 months, while control group patients received a matching placebo. The primary endpoint in the analysis testing the efficacy of long-term post-procedural clopidogrel was a combined incidence of death, myocardial infarction, or stroke at 12 months.

At one year, long-term clopidogrel therapy was associated with a 26.9% (3.9%–44.4%) relative reduction in the primary endpoint, $p = 0.02$, compared to therapy with aspirin only. The absolute rate of the primary endpoint was 8.5% versus 11.5% in the clopidogrel and placebo groups, respectively. Both the rates of death (1.7% versus 2.3%) and myocardial infarction (6.7% versus 8.4%) were numerically lower in the clopidogrel group (although not statistically significantly different). Likewise, the rate of stroke was numerically lower in the clopidogrel group (0.9% versus 1.1%, $p = \text{NS}$).

In summary, therapy with clopidogrel for up to one year after PCI was associated with a lower rate of adverse ischemic events. There was also a suggestion that clopidogrel loading with 300 mg may be associated with improved post-PCI outcome as long as the time interval between loading and the procedure is sufficiently long (in this trial at least six hours).

The PCI-Clopiodgrel as Adjunctive Reperfusion Therapy (CLARITY) trial analyzed a pre-specified subset of the patients who were treated with fibrinolysis for STEMI in the main CLARITY trial (see below). Patients were randomized to clopidogrel (300 mg load, followed by 75 mg daily) versus placebo with all patients receiving aspirin. Patients then underwent protocol-mandated coronary angiography two to eight days after randomization (median three days). A total of 1863 patients ended up undergoing PCI, and these patients were analyzed in the PCI-CLARITY trial with respect to clopidogrel pre-treatment.[51] The patients who were treated with a stent received open-label clopidogrel after PCI (with a loading dose administered in the catheterization laboratory). The primary endpoint was a composite of cardiovascular death, recurrent MI, or stroke between PCI and 30 days after randomization (Fig. 4). This was met in 3.6% of the pretreated patients versus 6.2% of the patients in the placebo group (adjusted OR 0.54 [0.35–0.85], $p = 0.008$). When this composite endpoint was analyzed from *randomization* to 30 days (thus capturing the pre-PCI effect of the early clopidogrel therapy as well), the event rates were 7.5% versus 12.0% for clopidogrel and placebo groups, respectively, adjusted OR 0.59 [0.43–0.81], $p = 0.001$. Importantly, there was no increase in bleeding. Thrombolysis in Myocardial Infarction (TIMI) major or minor bleeding rates for clopidogrel and placebo groups were 2.0% and 1.9%, respectively, $p > 0.99$.

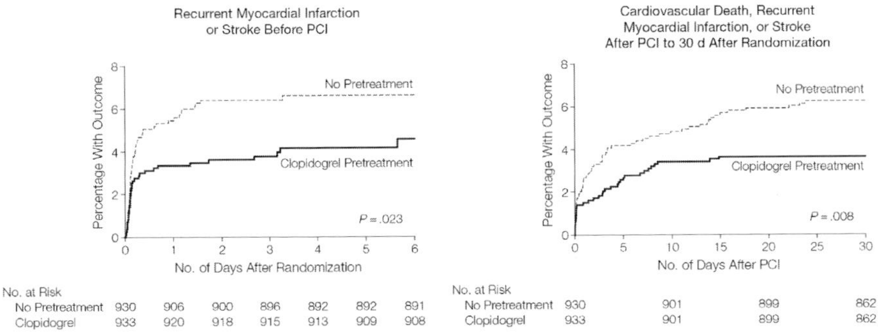

Fig. 4. Incidence of cardiovascular endpoints before and after percutaneous coronary intervention in the PCI-CLARITY trial (reprinted with permission from *JAMA*).

These data strongly argue for the early use of clopidogrel in STEMI and for clopidogrel pre-treatment in PCI.

The rupture of a coronary artery atherosclerotic plaque, followed by the interplay of platelet aggregation and the activation of the coagulation cascade, leads to the thrombotic occlusion of the epicardial coronary artery. This pathophysiology of the acute ST-elevation myocardial infarction clearly identifies the platelet as a major culprit. Although, the main therapy is reperfusion with either administration of a fibrinolytic agent or mechanical reperfusion via primary percutaneous coronary intervention, adjunctive pharmacotherapies remain critically important. These include aspirin in all cases, and intravenous platelet glycoprotein IIb/IIIa receptor inhibitors in the case of primary PCI. It is therefore reasonable to postulate that clopidogrel with its antiplatelet and perhaps anti-inflammatory action might also improve outcomes in acute ST-elevation myocardial infarction.

In the case of primary PCI, most procedures involve placement of intracoronary stents, and thus the same considerations apply as discussed with elective/urgent PCI. Clearly, there is less time to achieve clopidogrel loading as the procedure is unanticipated. No randomized trial data exist in the setting of primary PCI, but it is probably reasonable to administer a clopidogrel loading dose upon the decision to pursue primary PCI. Alternatively, a more conservative approach would be to forgo the benefits of clopidogrel loading (albeit with less than optimal duration of loading) and withhold clopidogrel until the coronary anatomy is delineated and until it is clear that the patient is not developing mechanical complications of acute

ST-elevation myocardial infarction that might require emergent open heart surgery. However, only 4%–6% of patients require CABG. Thus, it is less of an issue and early clopidogrel therapy is likely the optimal strategy.

Adjunctive pharmacotherapy in the setting of administration of fibrinolytic agents for acute ST-elevation myocardial infarction includes aspirin and intravenous unfractionated heparin.[52,53] Recently, two trials have tested the safety and efficacy of dual antiplatelet therapy with aspirin plus clopidogrel in this setting. Clopidogrel as Adjunctive Reperfusion Therapy (CLARITY) — TIMI-28 trial randomized 3491 patients with acute ST-elevation myocardial infarction (being treated with fibrinolytic therapy, aspirin, and heparin) to clopidogrel versus placebo.[54] Clopidogrel was administered as a loading dose of 300 mg, followed by daily dose of 75 mg. All patients were scheduled to undergo coronary angiography two to eight days after administration of the fibrinolytic agent. The primary endpoint of the study was an occluded infarct-related coronary artery on angiography with death or myocardial infarction before angiography as surrogates of an occluded artery. The patients who received clopidogrel had a lower incidence of the primary endpoint compared to patients who received a placebo: 15.0% versus 21.7%, respectively, $p = 0.00036$. This represented an odds reduction of 36%, and was largely driven by the lower rate of angiographic occlusion in the clopidogrel group. The 30-day incidence of the combined endpoint of cardiovascular death, recurrent myocardial infarction, or need for urgent revascularization was lower in the clopidogrel group compared to the control group: 11.6% versus 14.1%, respectively, $p = 0.03$, corresponding to a 20% odds reduction. Major bleeding was similar between the two groups (1.3% versus 1.1%, $p = 0.64$). This was true even among patients going on to CABG and those whose CABG took place within five days of clopidogrel therapy. Based on these data, clopidogrel appears to be a beneficial adjunct to fibrinolytic therapy, heparin, and aspirin in the management of acute STEMI.

The Clopidogrel Metoprolol Myocardial Infarction Trial/Second Chinese Cardiac Study (COMMIT/CCS2) was the second largest trial that has ever evaluated the therapy of acute myocardial infarction.[55,56] The two-by-two factorial designed study randomized over 45,000 patients with acute STEMI to clopidogrel 75 mg versus placebo (all patients received aspirin). The other comparison was between metoprolol versus placebo. The study was conducted in China and background therapy included aspirin. A 7% relative risk reduction was observed with clopidogrel therapy in the risk of in-hospital death (7.5% versus 8.1%, $p = 0.03$). A similar 9% relative risk reduction was noted in the short-term combined endpoint of death, recurrent myocardial infarction, or stroke, as well (9.3% versus 10.1%, $p = 0.002$). Of note, bleeding complications were similar in the two groups, with no increase in intracranial hemorrhage.

These two trials together provide data showing that the addition of clopidogrel to standard treatment for STEMI improves infarct related artery patency, reduces ischemic complications, and reduces mortality without any increase in bleeding. It can thus be added to current treatment algorithms for fibrinolytic and medical therapy for STEMI.

Considerations with Percutaneous Coronary Intervention

Most coronary angioplasty procedures involve the implantation of one or more intracoronary stents. The most devastating complication following stent placement is thrombosis within that stent, leading to transmural myocardial infarction. Clopidogrel markedly reduces the incidence of acute stent thrombosis in the time period when the stent is not yet endothelialized. With bare metal stents this process starts to occur within one month after stent placement. However, in the case of drug-eluting stents, the endothelialization process is delayed, and it is not clear when it is safe to discontinue clopidogrel therapy. Recently, several cases of stent thrombosis have been observed upon discontinuation of clopidogrel years after the placement of a drug-eluting stent.[57] Bavry and colleagues meta-analyzed 14 drug-eluting stent versus bare metal stent trials and discovered a higher incidence of late (>1 year) stent thrombosis among the patients who were treated with a drug-eluting stent.[58] Following the discontinuation of clopidogrel, patients in the Basel Stent Kosten Effektivitats Trial (BASKET) who had been treated with a drug-eluting stent were more likely to suffer a cardiac death or myocardial infarction compared to the patients who were treated with a bare metal stent.[59] Another analysis by Eisenstein *et al.* revealed that extended use of clopidogrel among patients who had received drug-eluting stents was associated with a lower risk of death.[60] Therefore, many interventional cardiologists prefer to maintain clopidogrel therapy indefinitely after drug-eluting stent placement, provided that the patient is tolerating it well.[61,62]

It is clear that undergoing percutaneous coronary intervention in the setting of adequate clopidogrel pretreatment is associated with a lower incidence of post-procedural adverse ischemic outcomes compared to inadequate pretreatment.[63,64] In fact, some evidence suggests that clopidogrel pretreatment may obviate the need for the use of platelet glycoprotein IIb/IIIa inhibitor agents in low-risk elective PCI. The Intracoronary Stenting and Antithrombotic Regimen — Rapid Early Action for Coronary Treatment (ISAR REACT) trial randomized 2159 patients undergoing low-risk elective coronary angioplasty who had been pretreated with clopidogrel (600 mg loading dose at least two hours prior to the procedure) to abciximab versus placebo and demonstrated a similar incidence of major adverse cardiac events (4% versus 4%, for abciximab versus placebo, respectively, relative risk with abciximab 1.05 (0.69–1.59, $p = 0.82$).[65] A similar result was noted in the Intracoronary Stenting and Antithrombotic Regimen — Is Abciximab a Superior Way to Eliminate Elevated Thrombotic Risk in Diabetics (ISAR-SWEET) trial.[66] In that trial a total of 701 diabetics undergoing elective PCI with stenting (with identical clopidogrel pretreatment regimen as in ISAR-REACT) were randomized to receive abciximab versus placebo, and similar incidence of death or myocardial infarction was observed at one year following the PCI in the two groups (8.3% versus 8.6%, $p = 0.91$). However, it appears that *troponin-positive* patients undergoing PCI for *acute coronary syndrome* do benefit from platelet glycoprotein IIb/IIIa inhibitor agents. This finding was observed in the ISAR REACT-2 trial, in which after clopidogrel loading, patients randomized to abciximab had fewer adverse events compared to the placebo group (8.9% versus 11.9%, $p = 0.03$).[67]

It appears that a 600 mg clopidogrel loading dose should be administered at least two hours before PCI in order to perform the procedure under conditions of maximal platelet inhibition.[68] Findings from the CREDO trial would suggest that the minimum time interval between a 300 mg clopidogrel loading dose and PCI associated with a clinical benefit may be as long as 12 hours. Practically, many interventional cardiologists administer a clopidogrel loading dose as soon as they think that angioplasty will likely take place (provided that there are no contraindications).

There is growing interest in higher loading doses achieving more rapid platelet inhibition. The study by Muller and colleagues demonstrated that clopidogrel loading with a dose of 600 mg achieved the steady-state level of ADP-induced platelet aggregation inhibition sooner than did 300 mg loading dose.[68] In the Clopidogrel Loading with Eptifibatide to Arrest the Reactivity of Platelets (CLEAR PLATELETS) study examining clopidogrel loading immediately following elective PCI with stenting, Gurbel *et al.* demonstrated that a 600 mg dose suppresses ADP-induced platelet aggregation more rapidly compared to a 300 mg dose.[69] A report by Zidar and colleagues also noted the more rapid inhibition of ADP-induced platelet aggregation with a 600 mg compared to a 300 mg loading dose in healthy volunteers (crossover design);[70] interestingly, the higher loading dose also more effectively suppressed the expression of platclet inflammatory markers.

In the Antiplatelet therapy for Reduction of MYocardial Damage during Angioplasty (ARMYDA)-2 trial, 255 patients undergoing PCI were randomized to 600 mg versus 300 mg clopidogrel loading dose administered four to eight hours before the procedure.[71] The incidence of the primary composite endpoint of death, myocardial infarction, and target vessel revascularization through 30 days was lower among the patients receiving the 600 mg loading dose. This was due entirely to reduction in post-PCI myocardial infarction (4.0% versus 11.6%, $p < 0.05$). The Intracoronary Stenting and Antithrombotic Regimen: Choose between three High Oral doses for Immediate Clopidogrel Effect (ISAR-CHOICE) trial evaluated clopidogrel loading doses of 300, 600, and 900 mg among 60 patients undergoing coronary angiography.[72] Loading with the 600 mg dose resulted in higher concentrations of clopidogrel and lower levels of platelet aggregation compared to the 300 mg dose. There was no additional inhibition of platelet function with the 900 mg dose. The Assessment of the best Loading dose of clopidogrel to Blunt platelet activation, Inflammation, and Ongoing Necrosis (ALBION) trial evaluated three different clopidogrel loading doses (300 versus 600 versus 900 mg; all patients received maintenance dose of 75 mg daily thereafter) in 103 patients undergoing PCI in the setting of a non-ST-elevation acute coronary syndrome.[73] The patients in the 600 and 900 mg groups achieved more rapid platelet inhibition compared to the patients in the control group (300 mg). Of note, there were no differences across the groups in the levels of inflammatory markers. These data in total suggest that clopidogrel loading doses higher than the routinely used 300 mg may be more effective in lowering the incidence of ischemic events in patients undergoing PCI. However, more work is required to determine the optimal pre-PCI loading regimen for clopidogrel.

In a study that included 20 patients on maintenance clopidogrel therapy for $\geq$ 1 month, the administration of a clopidogrel dose of 600 mg yielded further inhibition of ADP-induced platelet aggregation (from 52% aggregation to 33% aggregation).[74] An observation from PCI CLARITY was that even among patients who had been pretreated, those who were reloaded in the catheterization laboratory had lower event rates. The full meaning of this intriguing finding has not been determined as the efficacy and safety of a clopidogrel re-loading dose requires further investigation.

Novel Oral ADP Receptor Antagonists

Prasugrel (CS-747, LY640315), a novel oral $P2Y_{12}$ antagonist, was recently evaluated in the Joint Utilization of Medications to Block Platelets Optimally — Thrombolysis in Myocardial Infarction-26 (JUMBO-TIMI-26) trial.[75] Preclinical studies had showed that prasugrel had greater potency and more rapid onset of action (perhaps as a result of more rapid metabolism in blood) than did clopidogrel, setting the stage for a clinical trial. A total of 904 patients undergoing elective or urgent percutaneous coronary intervention were randomized to receive prasugrel (in three different dosing regimens) versus clopidogrel. All patients received 325 mg of aspirin. During the procedure, all patients received intravenous unfractionated heparin and the use of platelet glycoprotein IIb/IIIa receptor inhibitors was at the operator's discretion. The clopidogrel dosing regimen consisted of the clinically widely used 300 mg loading dose, followed by a daily dose of 75 mg. The three prasugrel regimens were 60 mg loading dose plus 15 mg daily (high dose), 60 mg plus 10 mg (intermediate dose), and 40 mg plus 7.5 mg (low dose). The primary endpoint of this phase-2 safety study was Thrombolysis in Myocardial Infarction (TIMI) minor plus major bleeding (excluding bleeding following coronary artery bypass graft surgery) in the first 30 days after PCI. The efficacy endpoints consisted of ischemic cardiac events through 30 days. Low rates of bleeding complications were observed in the two groups: the primary endpoint was 1.7% versus 1.2% among patients receiving prasugrel and clopidogrel, respectively, $p = 0.59$. Given the relatively low power of this trial, the confidence interval for the corresponding hazard ratio remains wide: 0.40–5.08. The rate of major adverse cardiac events through 30 days was similar in the two groups: 7.2% versus 9.4% among patients receiving prasugrel and clopidogrel, respectively, $p = 0.26$. In summary, this trial provided initial safety and efficacy data for prasugrel in contemporary PCI and sets the stage for the larger randomized trial designed to evaluate its efficacy in reducing ischemic adverse outcomes. This will be accomplished by the Trial to Assess Improvement in Therapeutic Outcomes by Optimizing Platelet Inhibition With Prasugrel (TRITON) — TIMI-38. Its design calls for a randomization of an estimated 13,000 patients presenting with an acute coronary syndrome (including STEMI) and a plan to proceed with early invasive strategy with heart catheterization and possible PCI to receive prasugrel versus clopidogrel for a median of 12 months. All patients will also receive aspirin. The primary endpoint will be a composite of cardiovascular death, myocardial infarction, and stroke.

AZD6140, which is currently under development as a novel oral $P2Y_{12}$ antagonist, is the first reversible oral ADP receptor antagonist. It is not a thienopyridine, but instead belongs to a class of medications called cyclopentyl-triazolo-pyrimidines (CPTP). It is biologically active without requiring activation by a liver cytochrome, giving it a rapid onset of action. Early experiments suggest that it blocks platelet activation and aggregation more consistently and completely than clopidogrel. The DISPERSE2–TIMI-33 trial evaluated AZD6140 at two doses (either 90 mg twice daily or 180 mg twice daily) versus clopidogrel 75 mg daily for up to 12 weeks in 990 patients with a non-ST elevation acute coronary syndrome. All patients also received aspirin. The primary endpoint was a composite of major and minor bleeding and it was similar in the three groups (10.2% for each of the AZD6140 groups versus 9.2% for the clopidogrel group).[76]

The role of the $P2Y_1$ receptor in thrombin-dependent tissue factor-induced thromboembolism was investigated in a series of experiments by Léon and colleagues. They administered intravenous human thromboplastin to wild-type and $P2Y_1$-knockout mice and detected a resistance to thromboembolism in the $P2Y_1$-deficient mice only.[77] The investigators also demonstrated the importance of the $P2Y_1$ receptor by documenting similar effect as seen with the knock-out mouse, with the selective antagonist of the $P2Y_1$ receptor (N^6-methyl-2′-deoxyadenosine-3′:5′-bisphosphate) on wild-type mice. An experimental agent MRS2179, a $P2Y_1$ receptor antagonist, is currently under investigation. Another target that to date has not been clinically utilized is the $P2X_1$ receptor.

Intravenous ADP Receptor Antagonists

Cangrelor (AR-C69931MX) is a highly potent and selective reversible $P2Y_{12}$ receptor antagonist (Fig. 5). It is an ATP analogue with a molecular weight of 800 Daltons. Unlike clopidogrel, it is active *in vitro*. With a mean half-life of 2.6 minutes, it is suitable for intravenous administration. Testing has demonstrated the return of platelet aggregation to pre-infusion levels within 20 minutes of the discontinuation of infusion. At an infusion rate of 4 mcg/kg/minute it inhibits over 90% of platelet aggregation. A phase-2 safety study of cangrelor in 39 patients with an acute coronary syndrome receiving treatment with aspirin, heparin, and nitrates revealed that although some bleeding was common (noted in 56% of patients), there were no instances of TIMI major or minor bleeding.[78]

In another evaluation, cangrelor was compared to placebo among 91 patients with a non-ST elevation acute coronary syndrome receiving aspirin and a heparinoid.[79] In this study, the incidence of bleeding complications was higher in the cangrelor group compared to the placebo group: 38% versus 26% (p-value not reported). On the other hand, an evaluation of

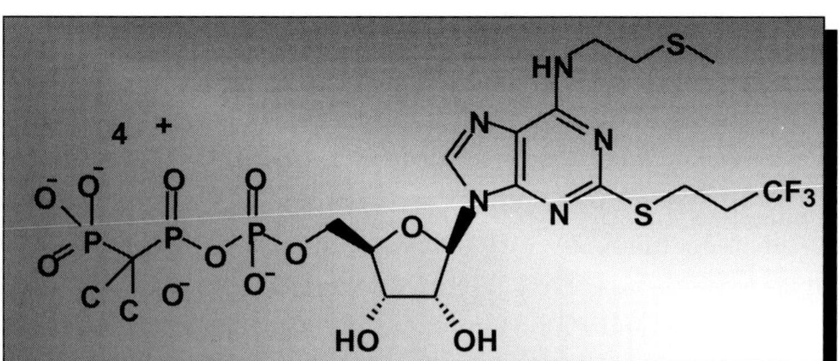

Fig. 5. The molecular structure of cangrelor.

cangrelor in 200 patients undergoing percutaneous coronary intervention did not demonstrate an elevated bleeding rate compared with abciximab.[80] Cangrelor was also studied as an adjunctive antiplatelet therapy in the fibrinolytic treatment of acute ST elevation myocardial infarction.[81] In this trial of 101 patients, the rates of ischemic adverse events and bleeding complications through 30 days, and TIMI grade-3 flow in the epicardial culprit coronary artery were similar in the cangrelor and control groups.

There are two ongoing phase-3 trials: Cangrelor versus standard tHerapy to Achieve optimal Management of Platelet InhibitiON (CHAMPION) PCI and CHAMPION PLATFORM.

Future Directions

The Clopidogrel for High Atherothrombotic Risk and Ischemic Stabilization, Management, and Avoidance (CHARISMA) trial of 15,603 patients evaluated clopidogrel 75 mg versus placebo among high-risk patients receiving aspirin.[82] Inclusion criteria required one of the following high-risk features: coronary artery disease, peripheral vascular disease, cerebrovascular disease, or risk factors for atherothrombosis. There was no difference between the comparator groups in the primary endpoint, a composite of cardiovascular death, myocardial infarction, and stroke (6.8% versus 7.3%, $p = 0.22$), or in severe bleeding (1.7% versus 1.3%, $p = 0.09$). Of note, among the 12,153 patients with documented cardiovascular disease, the patients who received clopidogrel plus aspirin had a lower incidence of the primary endpoint: 6.9% versus 7.9%, $p = 0.046$. In particular, patients with prior myocardial infarction, prior ischemic stroke, or symptomatic peripheral arterial disease appeared to benefit.

The Atrial Fibrillation Clopidogrel Trials with Irbesartan for prevention of Vascular Events (ACTIVE) trial is in the process of randomizing 14,500 patients with atrial fibrillation to irbesartan versus placebo. Those patients who are not deemed to be willing or able to take a vitamin K antagonist are additionally being randomized to clopidogrel (75 mg daily) versus placebo with all patients receiving concomitant aspirin. On the other hand, patients who are candidates for warfarin were being randomized to clopidogrel plus aspirin versus warfarin targeting an international normalized ratio of two to three (of note, this group will not receive aspirin). However, this part of the trial has been discontinued early due to an interim finding of a significant benefit favoring the anticoagulation arm. The patients in the other two parts of the trial will receive therapy for a planned two to four years. It thus appears based on preliminary data that anticoagulation is superior to dual antiplatelet therapy in the treatment of atrial fibrillation.

Summary

Clopidogrel reduces ischemic complications across a wide range of atherothrombotic disease and is relatively safe with respect to both bleeding and hematologic adverse events. Given its benefits, yet relatively modest level of platelet inhibition, it is possible that either more potent ADP receptor antagonists or higher doses of clopidogrel may provide greater clinical benefit. This hypothesis that "more is better" is being tested in ongoing trials.

References

1. Hollopeter G, Jantzen HM, Vincent D, *et al.* Identification of the platelet ADP receptor targeted by antithrombotic drugs. *Nature* 2001;**409**:202–207.
2. Hass WK, Easton JD, Adams HP, Jr, *et al.* A randomized trial comparing ticlopidine hydrochloride with aspirin for the prevention of stroke in high-risk patients. Ticlopidine Aspirin Stroke Study Group. *N Engl J Med* 1989;**321**:501–507.
3. Gent M, Blakely JA, Easton JD, *et al.* The Canadian American Ticlopidine Study (CATS) in thromboembolic stroke. *Lancet* 1989;**1**:1215–1220.
4. Gorelick PB, Richardson D, Kelly M, *et al.* Aspirin and ticlopidine for prevention of recurrent stroke in black patients: a randomized trial. *JAMA* 2003;**289**:2947–2957.
5. Balsano F, Rizzon P, Violi F, *et al.* Antiplatelet treatment with ticlopidine in unstable angina. A controlled multicenter clinical trial. The Studio della Ticlopidina nell'Angina Instabile Group. *Circulation* 1990;**82**:17–26.
6. Hall P, Nakamura S, Maiello L, *et al.* A randomized comparison of combined ticlopidine and aspirin therapy versus aspirin therapy alone after

successful intravascular ultrasound-guided stent implantation. *Circulation* 1996;**93**:215–222.

7. Schomig A, Neumann FJ, Kastrati A, *et al.* A randomized comparison of antiplatelet and anticoagulant therapy after the placement of coronary-artery stents. *N Engl J Med* 1996;**334**:1084–1089.
8. Urban P, Macaya C, Rupprecht HJ, *et al.* Randomized evaluation of anticoagulation versus antiplatelet therapy after coronary stent implantation in high-risk patients: the multicenter aspirin and ticlopidine trial after intracoronary stenting (MATTIS). *Circulation* 1998;**98**:2126–2132.
9. Leon MB, Baim DS, Popma JJ, *et al.* A clinical trial comparing three antithrombotic-drug regimens after coronary-artery stenting. Stent Anticoagulation Restenosis Study Investigators. *N Engl J Med* 1998;**339**:1665–1671.
10. Bertrand ME, Legrand V, Boland J, *et al.* Randomized multicenter comparison of conventional anticoagulation versus antiplatelet therapy in unplanned and elective coronary stenting. The full anticoagulation versus aspirin and ticlopidine (fantastic) study. *Circulation* 1998;**98**:1597–1603.
11. Limet R, David JL, Magotteaux P, *et al.* Prevention of aorta-coronary bypass graft occlusion. Beneficial effect of ticlopidine on early and late patency rates of venous coronary bypass grafts: a double-blind study. *J Thorac Cardiovasc Surg* 1987;**94**:773–783.
12. Chevigne M, David JL, Rigo P, Limet R. Effect of ticlopidine on saphenous vein bypass patency rates: a double-blind study. *Ann Thorac Surg* 1984;**37**:371–378.
13. Janzon L, Bergqvist D, Boberg J, *et al.* Prevention of myocardial infarction and stroke in patients with intermittent claudication; effects of ticlopidine. Results from STIMS, the Swedish Ticlopidine Multicentre Study. *J Intern Med* 1990;**227**:301–308.
14. Bergqvist D, Almgren B, Dickinson JP. Reduction of requirement for leg vascular surgery during long-term treatment of claudicant patients with ticlopidine: results from the Swedish Ticlopidine Multicentre Study (STIMS). *Eur J Vasc Endovasc Surg* 1995;**10**:69–76.
15. Becquemin JP. Effect of ticlopidine on the long-term patency of saphenous-vein bypass grafts in the legs. Etude de la Ticlopidine apres Pontage Femoro-Poplite and the Association Universitaire de Recherche en Chirurgie. *N Engl J Med* 1997;**337**:1726–1731.
16. Arcan JC, Blanchard J, Boissel JP, *et al.* Multicenter double-blind study of ticlopidine in the treatment of intermittent claudication and the prevention of its complications. *Angiology* 1988;**39**:802–811.

17. Balsano F, Coccheri S, Libretti A, *et al.* Ticlopidine in the treatment of intermittent claudication: a 21-month double-blind trial. *J Lab Clin Med* 1989;**114**:84–91.
18. Antiplatelet Trialists' Collaboration. Collaborative overview of randomised trials of antiplatelet therapy–I. Prevention of death, myocardial infarction, and stroke by prolonged antiplatelet therapy in various categories of patients. *BMJ* 1994;**308**:81–106.
19. Yeh SP, Hsueh EJ, Wu H, Wang YC. Ticlopidine-associated aplastic anemia. A case report and review of literature. *Ann Hematol* 1998;**76**:87–90.
20. Bennett CL, Davidson CJ, Raisch DW, *et al.* Thrombotic thrombocytopenic purpura associated with ticlopidine in the setting of coronary artery stents and stroke prevention. *Arch Intern Med* 1999;**159**:2524–2528.
21. Orford JL, Fasseas P, Melby S, *et al.* Safety and efficacy of aspirin, clopidogrel, and warfarin after coronary stent placement in patients with an indication for anticoagulation. *Am Heart J* 2004;**147**:463–467.
22. Saw J, Steinhubl SR, Berger PB, *et al.* Lack of adverse clopidogrel-atorvastatin clinical interaction from secondary analysis of a randomized, placebo-controlled clopidogrel trial. *Circulation* 2003;**108**:921–924.
23. Bates ER, Lau WC, Bleske BE. Loading, pretreatment, and interindividual variability issues with clopidogrel dosing. *Circulation* 2005;**111**:2557–2559.
24. Rajagopal V, Bhatt DL. Controversies of oral antiplatelet therapy in acute coronary syndromes and percutaneous coronary intervention. *Semin Thromb Hemost* 2004;**30**:649–655.
25. Quinn MJ, Bhatt DL, Zidar F, *et al.* Effect of clopidogrel pretreatment on inflammatory marker expression in patients undergoing percutaneous coronary intervention. *Am J Cardiol* 2004;**93**:679–684.
26. Vivekananthan DP, Bhatt DL, Chew DP, *et al.* Effect of clopidogrel pretreatment on periprocedural rise in C-reactive protein after percutaneous coronary intervention. *Am J Cardiol* 2004;**94**:358–360.
27. Mehta SR, McQueen MJ, Smieja M, *et al.* Baseline high-sensitivity C-reactive protein offers prognostic value in addition to contemporary risk stratification in non-ST-segment elevation acute coronary syndrome: results from the CURE inflammatory marker substudy (abstract). *Circulation* 2004;**110**:III–499 (abstract 2343).
28. Beinart SC, Kolm P, Veledar E, *et al.* Long-term cost effectiveness of early and sustained dual oral antiplatelet therapy with clopidogrel given for up to one year after percutaneous coronary intervention results: from the Clopidogrel for the Reduction of Events During Observation (CREDO) trial. *J Am Coll Cardiol* 2005;**46**:761–769.

29. Weintraub WS, Mahoney EM, Lamy A, *et al.* Long-term cost-effectiveness of clopidogrel given for up to one year in patients with acute coronary syndromes without ST-segment elevation. *J Am Coll Cardiol* 2005;**45**:838–845.
30. CAPRIE Steering Committee. A randomised, blinded, trial of clopidogrel versus aspirin in patients at risk of ischaemic events (CAPRIE). *Lancet* 1996;**348**:1329–1339.
31. Cannon CP. Effectiveness of clopidogrel versus aspirin in preventing acute myocardial infarction in patients with symptomatic atherothrombosis (CAPRIE trial). *Am J Cardiol* 2002;**90**:760–762.
32. Bhatt DL, Chew DP, Hirsch AT, *et al.* Superiority of clopidogrel versus aspirin in patients with prior cardiac surgery. *Circulation* 2001;**103**:363–368.
33. Ringleb PA, Bhatt DL, Hirsch AT, *et al.* Benefit of clopidogrel over aspirin is amplified in patients with a history of ischemic events. *Stroke* 2004;**35**:528–532.
34. Bhatt DL, Marso SP, Hirsch AT, *et al.* Amplified benefit of clopidogrel versus aspirin in patients with diabetes mellitus. *Am J Cardiol* 2002;**90**:625–628.
35. Bhatt DL, Hirsch AT, Ringleb PA, *et al.* Reduction in the need for hospitalization for recurrent ischemic events and bleeding with clopidogrel instead of aspirin. CAPRIE investigators. *Am Heart J* 2000;**140**:67–73.
36. Caro JJ, Migliaccio-Walle K. Generalizing the results of clinical trials to actual practice: the example of clopidogrel therapy for the prevention of vascular events. CAPRA (CAPRIE Actual Practice Rates Analysis) Study Group. Clopidogrel versus aspirin in patients at risk of ischaemic events. *Am J Med* 1999;**107**:568–572.
37. Diener HC, Bogousslavsky J, Brass LM, *et al.* Aspirin and clopidogrel compared with clopidogrel alone after recent ischaemic stroke or transient ischaemic attack in high-risk patients (MATCH): randomised, double-blind, placebo-controlled trial. *Lancet* 2004;**364**:331–337.
38. Markus HS, Droste DW, Kaps M, *et al.* Dual antiplatelet therapy with clopidogrel and aspirin in symptomatic carotid stenosis evaluated using doppler embolic signal detection: the Clopidogrel and Aspirin for Reduction of Emboli in Symptomatic Carotid Stenosis (CARESS) trial. *Circulation* 2005;**111**:2233–2240.
39. Hankey GJ. Ongoing and planned trials of antiplatelet therapy in the acute and long-term management of patients with ischaemic brain syndromes: setting a new standard of care. *Cerebrovasc Dis* 2004;**17**(Suppl 3):11–16.
40. Royal College of Physicians. *National Clinical Guidelines for Stroke*, 2nd ed. (2004). Accessed via www.strokecenter.org/prof/guidelines.htm on 10/28/2005.

41. Bertrand ME, Rupprecht HJ, Urban P, *et al.* Double-blind study of the safety of clopidogrel with and without a loading dose in combination with aspirin compared with ticlopidine in combination with aspirin after coronary stenting: The Clopidogrel Aspirin Stent International Cooperative Study (CLASSICS). *Circulation* 2000;**102**:624–629.
42. Bhatt DL, Bertrand ME, Berger PB, *et al.* Meta-analysis of randomized and registry comparisons of ticlopidine with clopidogrel after stenting. *J Am Coll Cardiol* 2002;**39**:9–14.
43. Yusuf S, Zhao F, Mehta SR, *et al.* Effects of clopidogrel in addition to aspirin in patients with acute coronary syndromes without ST-segment elevation. *N Engl J Med* 2001;**345**:494–502.
44. Peters RJ, Mehta SR, Fox KA, *et al.* Effects of aspirin dose when used alone or in combination with clopidogrel in patients with acute coronary syndromes: observations from the Clopidogrel in Unstable angina to prevent Recurrent Events (CURE) study. *Circulation* 2003;**108**:1682–1687.
45. Hirsh J, Bhatt DL. Comparative benefits of clopidogrel and aspirin in high-risk patient populations: lessons from the CAPRIE and CURE studies. *Arch Intern Med* 2004;**164**:2106–2110.
46. Budaj A, Yusuf S, Mehta SR, *et al.* Benefit of clopidogrel in patients with acute coronary syndromes without ST-segment elevation in various risk groups. *Circulation* 2002;**106**:1622–1626.
47. Mehta SR, Yusuf S, Peters RJ, *et al.* Effects of pretreatment with clopidogrel and aspirin followed by long-term therapy in patients undergoing percutaneous coronary intervention: the PCI-CURE study. *Lancet* 2001;**358**: 527–533.
48. Yusuf S, Mehta SR, Zhao F, *et al.* Early and late effects of clopidogrel in patients with acute coronary syndromes. *Circulation* 2003;**107**:966–972.
49. The Clopidogrel in Unstable Angina to Prevent Recurrent Events Trial Investigators. Effects of clopidogrel in addition to aspirin in patients with acute coronary syndromes without ST-segment elevation. *N Engl J Med* 2001;**345**:494–502.
50. Steinhubl SR, Berger PB, Mann JT, *et al.* Early and sustained dual oral antiplatelet therapy following percutaneous coronary intervention: a randomized controlled trial. CREDO Investigators. *JAMA* 2002;**288**: 2411–2420.
51. Sabatine MS, Cannon CP, Gibson CM, *et al.* Effect of clopidogrel pretreatment before percutaneous coronary intervention in patients with ST-elevation myocardial infarction treated with fibrinolytics: the PCI-CLARITY study. *JAMA* 2005;**294**:1224–1232.

52. Fathi RB, Bhatt DL. Enhancing reperfusion therapy for myocardial infarction with dual antiplatelet therapy: breaking the glass ceiling. *Am Heart J* 2005;**149**:947–949.
53. Dogan A, Ozgul M, Ozaydin M, *et al.* Effect of clopidogrel plus aspirin on tissue perfusion and coronary flow in patients with ST-segment elevation myocardial infarction: a new reperfusion strategy. *Am Heart J* 2005;**149**:1037–1042.
54. Sabatine MS, Cannon CP, Gibson CM, *et al.* Addition of clopidogrel to aspirin and fibrinolytic therapy for myocardial infarction with ST-segment elevation. *N Engl J Med* 2005;**352**:1179–1189.
55. Chen ZM, Jiang LX, Chen YP, *et al.* Addition of clopidogrel to aspirin in 45,852 patients with acute myocardial infarction: randomised placebo-controlled trial. *Lancet* 2005;**366**:1607–1621.
56. Chen ZM, Pan HC, Chen YP, *et al.* Early intravenous then oral metoprolol in 45,852 patients with acute myocardial infarction: randomised placebo-controlled trial. *Lancet* 2005;**366**:1622–1632.
57. McFadden EP, Stabile E, Regar E, *et al.* Late thrombosis in drug-eluting coronary stents after discontinuation of antiplatelet therapy. *Lancet* 2004;**364**:1519–1521.
58. Bavry AA, Kumbhani DJ, Helton TJ, *et al.* Late thrombosis of drug-eluting stents: a meta-analysis of randomized clinical trials. *Am J Med* 2006;**119**:1056–1061.
59. Pfisterer M, Brunner-La Rocca HP, Buser PT, *et al.* Late clinical events after clopidogrel discontinuation may limit the benefit of drug-eluting stents: an observational study of drug-eluting versus bare-metal stents. *J Am Coll Cardiol* 2006;**48**:2584–2591.
60. Eisenstein EL, Anstrom KJ, Kong DF, *et al.* Clopidogrel use and long-term clinical outcomes after drug-eluting stent implantation. *JAMA* 2007;**297**:159–168.
61. Bavry AA, Kumbhani DJ, Helton TJ, Bhatt DL. Risk of thrombosis with the use of sirolimus-eluting stents for percutaneous coronary intervention (from registry and clinical trial data). *Am J Cardiol* 2005;**95**:1469–1472.
62. Bavry AA, Kumbhani DJ, Helton TJ, Bhatt DL. What is the risk of stent thrombosis associated with the use of paclitaxel-eluting stents for percutaneous coronary intervention? A meta-analysis. *J Am Coll Cardiol* 2005;**45**:941–946.
63. Chew DP, Bhatt DL, Robbins MA, *et al.* Effect of clopidogrel added to aspirin before percutaneous coronary intervention on the risk associated with C-reactive protein. *Am J Cardiol* 2001;**88**:672–674.
64. Chan AW, Moliterno DJ, Berger PB, *et al.* Triple antiplatelet therapy during percutaneous coronary intervention is associated with improved outcomes including one-year survival: results from the Do Tirofiban and

ReoProGive Similar Efficacy Outcome Trial (TARGET). *J Am Coll Cardiol* 2003;**42**:1188–1195.

65. Kastrati A, Mehilli J, Schuhlen H, *et al.* A clinical trial of abciximab in elective percutaneous coronary intervention after pretreatment with clopidogrel. *N Engl J Med* 2004;**350**:232–238.
66. Mehilli J, Kastrati A, Schuhlen H, *et al.* Randomized clinical trial of abciximab in diabetic patients undergoing elective percutaneous coronary interventions after treatment with a high loading dose of clopidogrel. *Circulation* 2004;**110**:3627–3635.
67. Kastrati A, Mehilli J, Neumann FJ, *et al.* Abciximab in patients with acute coronary syndromes undergoing percutaneous coronary intervention after clopidogrel pretreatment: the ISAR-REACT 2 randomized trial. *JAMA* 2006;**295**:1531–1538.
68. Muller I, Seyfarth M, Rudiger S, *et al.* Effect of a high loading dose of clopidogrel on platelet function in patients undergoing coronary stent placement. *Heart* 2001;**85**:92–93.
69. Gurbel PA, Bliden KP, Zaman KA, *et al.* Clopidogrel loading with eptifibatide to arrest the reactivity of platelets: results of the Clopidogrel Loading With Eptifibatide to Arrest the Reactivity of Platelets (CLEAR PLATELETS) study. *Circulation* 2005;**111**:1153–1159.
70. Zidar FJ, Moliterno DJ, Bhatt DL, *et al.* High dose clopidogrel loading rapidly reduces both platelet inflammatory marker expression and aggregation. *J Am Coll Cardiol* 2004;**43**(Suppl):64A.
71. Patti G, Colonna G, Pasceri V, *et al.* Randomized trial of high loading dose of clopidogrel for reduction of periprocedural myocardial infarction in patients undergoing coronary intervention: results from the ARMYDA-2 (Antiplatelet therapy for Reduction of MYocardial Damage during Angioplasty) study. *Circulation* 2005;**111**:2099–2106.
72. von Beckerath N, Taubert D, Pogatsa-Murray G, *et al.* Absorption, metabolization, and antiplatelet effects of 300-, 600-, and 900-mg loading doses of clopidogrel: results of the ISAR-CHOICE (Intracoronary Stenting and Antithrombotic Regimen: Choose Between 3 High Oral Doses for Immediate Clopidogrel Effect) Trial. *Circulation* 2005;**112**:2946–2950.
73. Montalescot G. Oral presentation at the Euro PCR conference (2005).
74. Kastrati A, von Beckerath N, Joost A, *et al.* Loading with 600 mg clopidogrel in patients with coronary artery disease with and without chronic clopidogrel therapy. *Circulation* 2004;**110**:1916–1919.
75. Wiviott SD, Antman EM, Winters KJ, *et al.* Randomized comparison of prasugrel (CS-747, LY640315), a novel thienopyridine P2Y12 antagonist,

with clopidogrel in percutaneous coronary intervention: results of the Joint Utilization of Medications to Block Platelets Optimally (JUMBO)-TIMI 26 trial. *Circulation* 2005;**111**:3366–3373.
76. Cannon CP, Husted S, Storey RF, *et al.* The DISPERSE 2 trial: safety, tolerability and preliminary efficacy of AZD6140, the first oral reversible ADP receptor antagonist, compared with clopidogrel in patients with non-ST segment elevation acute coronary syndrome. *Circulation* 2005;**112**:II–615 (abstract 2906).
77. Leon C, Freund M, Ravanat C, *et al.* Key role of the P2Y(1) receptor in tissue factor-induced thrombin-dependent acute thromboembolism: studies in P2Y(1)-knockout mice and mice treated with a P2Y(1) antagonist. *Circulation* 2001;**103**:718–723.
78. Storey RF, Oldroyd KG, Wilcox RG. Open multicentre study of the P2T receptor antagonist AR-C69931MX assessing safety, tolerability and activity in patients with acute coronary syndromes. *Thromb Haemost* 2001;**85**:401–407.
79. Jacobsson F, Swahn E, Wallentin L, Ellborg M. Safety profile and tolerability of intravenous AR-C69931MX, a new antiplatelet drug, in unstable angina pectoris and non-Q-wave myocardial infarction. *Clin Ther* 2002;**24**:752–765.
80. Weaver WD, Becker R, Harrington R, *et al.* Safety and efficacy of a novel direct P2T receptor antagonist, AR-C69931MX, in patients undergoing percutaneous coronary intervention. *Eur Heart J* 2000;**21**:382A.
81. Greenbaum AB, Ohman EM, Gibson MS, *et al.* Intravenous adenosine diphosphate P2T platelet receptor antagonism as an adjunct to fibrinolysis for acute myocardial infarction. *J Am Coll Cardiol* 2002;**39**:281A.
82. Bhatt DL, Fox KA, Hacke W, *et al.* Clopidogrel and aspirin versus aspirin alone for the prevention of atherothrombotic events. *N Engl J Med* 2006;**354**:1706–1717.

5 Monitoring Antiplatelet Therapy

Paul Harrison and Alan D. Michelson

Introduction

Platelets play a pivotal role in both normal hemostasis and pathological bleeding and thrombosis.[1] Most platelet function tests have been traditionally utilized for the diagnosis and management of patients presenting with bleeding problems rather than thrombosis.[2] However, as platelets are now implicated in the development of atherothrombosis, which is the leading cause of mortality in the Western world,[3,4] new and existing platelet function tests are increasingly being used for the monitoring the efficacy of the antiplatelet drugs to treat these conditions. This, coupled with the development of new, simpler tests and point-of-care (POC) instruments, has resulted in the increasing tendency of platelet function testing to be performed away from specialized hemostasis clinical or research laboratories, where the more traditional and complex tests are still performed.[5,6]

This chapter discusses currently available clinical tests for the monitoring of antiplatelet therapy. Table 1 is a summary of the currently available tests for the monitoring of antiplatelet therapy, including their advantages and disadvantages.

History of Platelet Function Testing and Overview of Currently Available Tests

Platelets were discovered in the 1880s.[7] Platelet function testing began with the application of the *in vivo* bleeding time by Duke in 1910.[8] The bleeding time was further refined by the Ivy technique and the availability

Table 1. An alphabetical list of currently available tests for the monitoring of antiplatelet therapy.

Name of test	Principle	Advantages	Disadvantages	Frequency of use
AspirinWorks®	Immunoassay of urinary 11-dehydro-thromboxane B_2	Measures stable thromboxane metabolite Dependent upon COX-1 activity	Indirect assay Not platelet-specific Renal function-dependent	Increasing use
Bleeding time	*In vivo* cessation of blood flow	*In vivo* test Physiological POC	Insensitive Invasive Scarring High CV	Decreasing popularity
Flow cytometry	Measurement of platelet glycoproteins and activation markers by fluorescence (e.g. VASP phosphorylation to monitor $P2Y_{12}$ inhibition)	Whole blood test Small blood volumes Wide variety of tests	Specialized operator Expensive Samples prone to artifact unless carefully prepared	Widely used
HemoStatus® device	Platelet procoagulant activity	Simple POC	Insensitive to aspirin and GPIb function	Used in surgery and cardiology
Ichor — Plateletworks®	Platelet counting pre- and post-activation	Rapid Simple POC Small blood volume	Indirect test measuring count after aggregation	Used in surgery and cardiology
Impact® cone and plate(let) analyzer	Quantification of high shear platelet adhesion/aggregation onto surface	Small blood volume required High shear Rapid Simple Research (variable) and fixed versions available POC	Instrument not yet widely available	Little widespread experience as only recently commercially available

(*Continued*)

Table 1. (*Continued*)

Name of test	Principle	Advantages	Disadvantages	Frequency of use
Light transmission aggregometry (LTA)	Low shear platelet-to-platelet aggregation in response to classical agonists	Gold standard	Time consuming Sample preparation Expensive	Widely used in specialized labs
PFA-100®	High shear platelet adhesion and aggregation during formation of a platelet plug	Whole blood test High shear Small blood volumes Simple Rapid POC	Inflexible VWF-dependent Hct-dependent Insensitive to clopidogrel	Widely used
Platelet reactivity index	Measurement of platelet aggregates in whole blood (modified Wu and Hoak method)	Simple Rapid Inexpensive	Requires blood counter Indirect test measuring count after aggregation	Little widespread experience
Serum thromboxane B_2	Immunoassay	Dependent upon COX-1 activity	Prone to artifact Not platelet-specific	Widespread use
Thromboelastography (TEG® or ROTEM®)	Monitoring of rate and quality of clot formation	Global whole blood test POC	Measures clot properties only; largely platelet-independent unless platelet activators are used	Used in surgery and anesthesiology
VerifyNow®	Fully automated platelet aggregometer to measure antiplatelet therapy	Simple POC 3 test cartridges (aspirin, $P2Y_{12}$ and GPIIb-IIIa)	Cartridges can only be used for single purpose	Increasing use

(*Continued*)

Table 1. (*Continued*)

Name of test	Principle	Advantages	Disadvantages	Frequency of use
Whole blood aggregometry	Monitors changes in impedance in response to classical agonists	Whole blood test	Older instruments require electrodes to be cleaned and recycled	Widely used in specialized labs although less than LTA

COX-1, cyclooxygenase-1; CV, coefficient of variation; GP, glycoprotein; Hct, hematocrit; LTA, light transmission aggregometry; PFA-100, platelet function analyzer-100; POC, point-of-care; VASP, vasodilator-stimulated phosphoprotein; VWF, von Willebrand factor.

of commercial spring-loaded template disposable devices containing sterile blades (e.g. Simplate II® from Organon Technika Corporation) and was still regarded as the most useful screening test of platelet function until the early 1990s.[2,9,10] In the last ten to 15 years, the widespread use of the bleeding time has rapidly declined because its limitations have been recognized (see below) and other, less invasive, screening tests have become available.[11–13]

Platelet aggregometry (light transmission aggregometry, LTA) was invented in the 1960s and soon revolutionized the identification and diagnosis of primary hemostatic defects.[14,15] LTA is still regarded as the gold standard of platelet function testing and by adding a panel of agonists at a range of concentrations to stirred platelets it is possible to obtain a large amount of information about many different aspects of platelet function and biochemistry.[16] This test, often now coupled with the measurement of stored and releasable platelet nucleotide content, is still utilized in most laboratories for the identification and diagnosis of many platelet defects.[17] Over more recent years, commercial aggregometers have become easier to use with multi-channel capability, simple automatic setting of 100% and 0% baselines, and computer operation and storage of results. For example, a new fully computerized eight-channel aggregometer has just become available (Fig. 1). Some instruments can simultaneously measure luminescence, to monitor the release reaction of dense granular nucleotides during secondary aggregation. Although still considered the most useful diagnostic and research tool, LTA is relatively non-physiological, as separated platelets are usually stirred under low shear conditions during the test and only form aggregates after addition of agonists, conditions which do not accurately

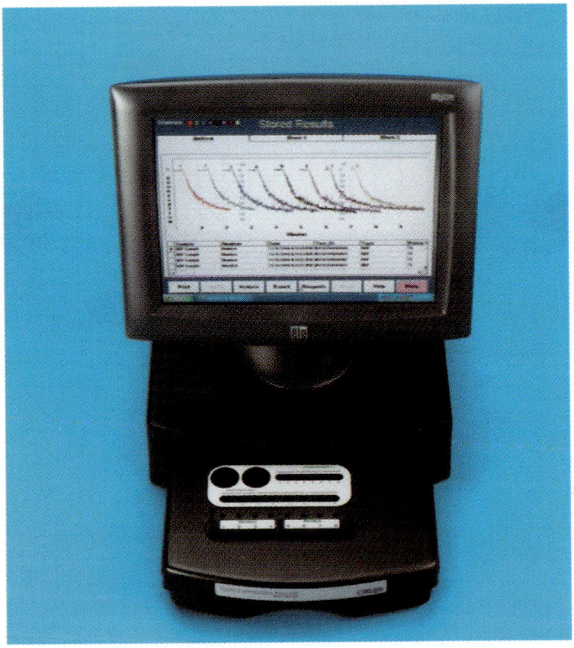

Fig. 1. An example of a modern eight-channel platelet aggregometer. The model shown is the Biodata PAP-8E®. Reproduced with permission from Biodata and Biodis.

mimic platelet adhesion, activation and aggregation upon vessel wall damage. Also conventional LTA using a full panel of agonists requires both large blood volumes and a significant expertise both to perform the tests and interpret the tracings. In response to the problems with the bleeding time and LTA, a number of alternative tests have been developed, including impedance whole blood aggregometry (WBA), a fully automated cartridge-based instrument (VerifyNow®) that measures platelet LTA in anticoagulated whole blood, and a variety of tests that attempt to simulate primary haemostasis *in vitro* (Table 1).

WBA provides a means to study platelet function within anticoagulated whole blood without any sample processing.[18] The test measures the change in resistance or impedance between two electrodes as platelets adhere and aggregate in response to classical agonists. The original instrument was a two-channel device with luminescence capability. A new fully computerized two- or four-channel instrument has now become available (Fig. 2).

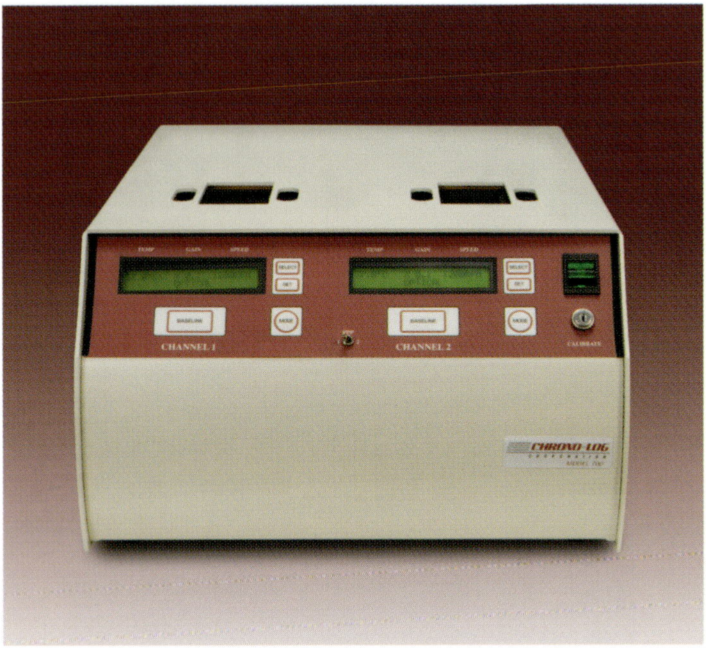

Fig. 2. The Chrono-log Model 700® whole blood/optical 2 channel lumiaggregometer. Reproduced with permission from Chrono-log.

Although the latter instrument can also be used for LTA of platelet-rich plasma (PRP), WBA has many significant advantages including the use of smaller sample volumes and the immediate analysis of samples without manipulation, loss of time or potential loss of platelet subpopulations or platelet activation during centrifugation. The main disadvantage of the older WBA instruments was that the electrodes had to be carefully cleaned to remove platelet aggregates after the test. However, disposable electrodes are now available. A new five-channel computerized WBA instrument (Multiple Platelet Function Analyzer or Multiplate®) has disposable cuvettes/electrodes with a range of different agonists for different applications including diagnosis and monitoring antiplatelet therapy.

The VerifyNow® (formerly known as the Ultegra Rapid Platelet Function Analyzer, RPFA) instrument (Fig. 3) is a fully automated POC test that was originally developed to monitor glycoprotein (GP) IIb-IIIa (integrin αIIbβ3) antagonists within a specialized self-contained cartridge

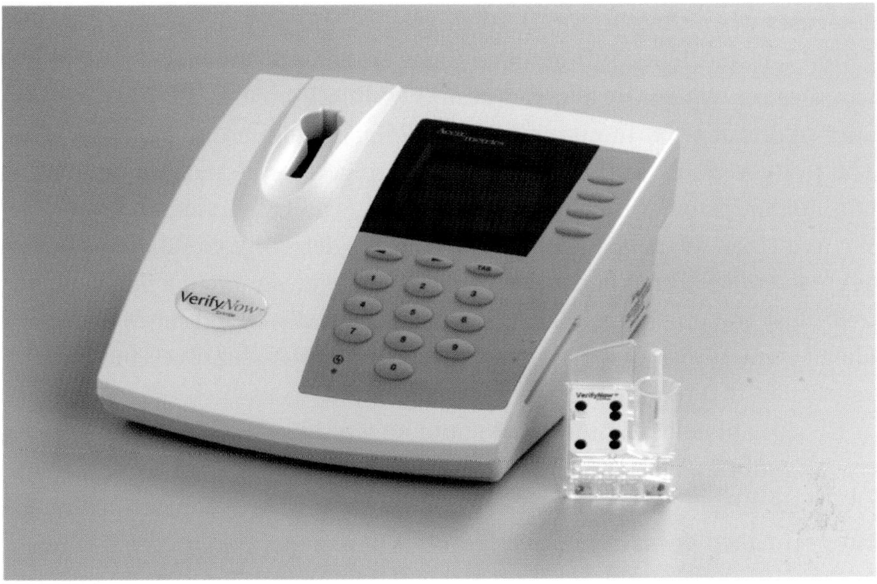

Fig. 3. The VerifyNow® system. Reproduced with permission from Accumetrics.

(containing a platelet activator and fibrinogen-coated beads) that is inserted into the instrument at test initiation.[19–21] Blood sample tubes are then simply mixed prior to insertion onto the cartridge that has been pre-mounted onto the instrument. Aggregation in response to the agonist is monitored by light transmission through two duplicate reaction chambers in each cartridge and the mean result displayed and printed after a few minutes. Other specialized cartridges are now available for measuring platelet responses to either aspirin (VerifyNow® Aspirin) or clopidogrel and other $P2Y_{12}$ antagonists (VerifyNow® P2Y12). This instrument is a considerable advance, as the test is a fully automated POC test without the requirements of sample transport, time delays or a specialized laboratory and it can provide immediate information. It is also relatively expensive. However, the test is specifically designed for monitoring three major classes of antiplatelet drugs.

It is also possible to monitor platelet aggregometry in whole blood by a simple platelet counting technique. After addition of an agonist to anticoagulated, stirred whole blood, platelets aggregate and the platelet count decreases when compared to a control tube.[22–24] The Plateletworks® aggregation kits and Ichor full blood counter (Helena Biosciences) are simply based upon comparing platelet counts within a control EDTA tube and after aggregation with either ADP or collagen within citrated tubes.[25–28] The test correlates well with standard aggregometry[29] and can be used to monitor antiplatelet therapy,[30,31] potentially as a POC device. In the 1970s, Wu and Hoak described a simple method for detecting circulating platelet aggregates.[32] This method was refined by Grotemeyer into the platelet reactivity test and compares platelet counts within two blood tubes anticoagulated with EDTA and EDTA/fixative. The EDTA dissolves the platelet aggregates that remain within the fixed sample.[33,34]

Because platelet LTA does not simulate physiological primary hemostasis, a number of tests have been developed that attempted to mimic the processes that occur during vessel wall damage. Many of these techniques have remained primarily research tools within expert laboratories because of their inherent complexity and technical difficulty. However, many simpler *in vitro* assays have been developed to measure platelet adhesion and retention of platelets on exposure to foreign surfaces. The original glass column platelet retention test was developed by Hellem.[35] Further modifications of this principle include the O'Brien filterometer,[36,37] the retention test Homburg[38,39] and the platelet adhesion assay (PADA).[40] More recently with significant advances in microscopy and digital imaging/processing it is now possible to perform real time imaging of fluorescently labeled platelets and coagulation system components during thrombus formation within animal models.[41–43] This has already resulted in some exciting new discoveries about platelets and the dynamics of their interaction with the vessel wall, each other and with the coagulation system. A number of prototype instruments have been developed over the years, some of which remained as research tools (e.g. Thrombotic Status Analyzer, TSA[44]) and some which were commercialized but are no longer available e.g. the Clot Signature Analyzer® (CSA) that was developed from the Haemostatometer.[45–47] Other commercially available instruments include the Platelet Function Analyzer-100 (PFA-100®, Fig. 4) and the Impact® cone and plate(let) analyzer. Both of these tests measure platelet adhesion and aggregation under conditions of high shear, in an attempt to simulate primary hemostatic mechanisms that are encountered *in vivo*.

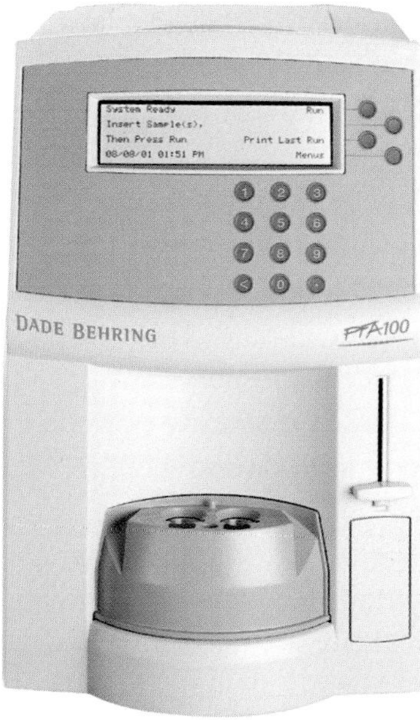

Fig. 4. The PFA-100® instrument. Reproduced with permission from Dade-Behring.

The cone and plate(let) analyzer was originally developed by Varon and monitors platelet adhesion and aggregation to a plate coated with collagen or extracellular matrix (ECM) under high shear conditions of 1800 s^{-1}.[48–50] In the commercial version of the device, the Impact® (DiaMed), a plastic plate is utilized instead of a collagen or an ECM-coated surface. The test is now fully automated, simple to operate, uses a small quantity of blood (0.12 ml) and displays results in six minutes. The instrument contains a microscope and performs staining and image analysis of the platelets that have adhered and aggregated on the plate. The software permits storage of the images from each analysis and records a number of parameters including surface coverage, average size and distribution histogram of adhered platelets. Preliminary data suggest the test can be used in the diagnosis of platelet defects and monitoring antiplatelet therapy. Because the test has only just become commercially available, widespread experience is limited. There is also a recently released research version of the instrument called the Impact-R that requires some of the test steps to be manually performed, but also facilitates adjustment of the shear rate.

The PFA-100® device has been available for a number of years and is now in widespread use within many laboratories with over 200 papers published on various clinical applications.[51,52] The test was originally developed as a prototype instrument called the Thrombostat-4000 by Kratzer and Born and further developed into the PFA-100® by Dade-Behring.[53,54] The PFA-100® measures the fall in flow rate as platelets within citrated whole blood are aspirated through a capillary and begin to seal a 150 μm aperture within a collagen-coated membrane. This reaction takes place contained within one of two types of disposable cartridge. The instrument records the time (closure time or CT) it takes to occlude the aperture, along with the total volume of blood used during the test. Maximal CTs that can be obtained are 300 seconds.

Platelets contribute significantly to the generation of thrombin and the dynamics of blood clotting including clot formation, clot retraction and lysis. Clot retraction can be easily measured in whole blood or PRP within glass tubes after the addition of calcium. The role of platelets in clot retraction was first described by Hayem in the late 19th century and Glanzmann famously described patients with poor clot retraction or thrombasthenia in 1918, who were subsequently shown to be defective in integrin αIIbβ3 (GPIIb-IIIa).[55] Modern tests are available that can study both the role of platelets in thrombin generation, clot formation and clot retraction. For example, thrombin generation tests can be used to measure thrombin generation in PRP and whole blood.[56–58] However, early tests involved subsampling and centrifugation steps to remove cells that would interfere with the measurement. The recent development of fluorescent thrombin substrates has enabled the test to be utilized in PRP and whole blood without the need for sub-sampling, and there is now commercially available software (Thrombinoscope®) that can be used to calculate the area under the thrombin generation curve, referred to as the endogenous thrombin potential (ETP). One company has developed a POC instrument that measures the influence of platelet activating factor on the kaolin activated clotting time. The HemoStatus® test (Medtronic Blood Management, Parker, CO, USA) can be used to detect the effects of GPIIb-IIIa antagonists.[59–61] There are also a number of instruments that measure the physical properties of clot formation. Thromboelastography® (TEG) was developed more than

50 years ago.[62–64] Anticoagulated whole blood is incubated in a heated sample cup in which a pin is suspended that is connected to a chart recorder or computer. The cup oscillates five degrees in each direction. In normal anticoagulated blood the pin is unaffected, but as the blood clots, the motion of the cup is transmitted to the pin. Whole blood or recalcified plasma can be used, with or without activators of the tissue factor or contact factor pathways. The instrument has been significantly upgraded to the TEG analyzer 5000 series. The TEG is relatively rapid to perform ($<$ 30 minutes), can be conducted in a POC fashion and provides various data relating to clot formation and lysis (the lag time before the clot starts to form, the rate at which clotting occurs, the maximal amplitude of the trace and the extent and rate of amplitude reduction). Rotational TEG (ROTEG® or ROTEM®) is an adaptation of the TEG in which the cup is stationary and the pin oscillates.[62,65] Unlike platelet function tests, TEG instruments have been traditionally utilized within surgical and anesthesiology departments as POC tests for determining the risk of bleeding and as a guide to transfusion requirements. More recent developments include an expansion in the range of activators to initiate aggregation rather than coagulation (e.g. the Platelet Mapping System® using ADP and arachidonic acid), making the Haemoscope TEG theoretically more sensitive to antiplatelet drugs than conventional TEG.[66,67] The Haemostasis Analysis System® (HAS) by Hemodyne is based upon the original technique developed by Carr.[68–71] The HAS® measures a number of parameters in clotting blood including platelet contractile force (PCF), clot elastic modulus and thrombin generation time (TGT) in a small sample (700 μl) of whole blood.

In the last 20 years, flow cytometric analysis of platelets has also developed into a powerful and popular means to study many aspects of platelet biology and function. Preferred modern methods now utilize diluted anticoagulated whole blood incubated with a variety of reagents including antibodies and dyes that bind specifically to individual platelet proteins, granules and lipid membranes.[72–74] Many of these reagents are now commercially available from many sources enabling flow cytometric analysis of platelets to be widely performed. Flow cytometric analysis of platelet function is discussed in detail in Refs. 72–74.

Monitoring Antiplatelet Therapy

Most platelet function tests have been traditionally utilized to either screen for or diagnose platelet defects. Most traditional tests are not only difficult to perform but are expensive, time consuming, and require relatively large volumes of fresh blood. They are therefore usually performed within specialized hemostasis laboratories, often in close proximity to their associated clinics. Many of these tests are limited in their capacity to predict bleeding or thrombosis. These limitations have largely restricted their widespread clinical use within other disciplines (e.g. cardiology, stroke and surgery). However, this is now beginning to change as simpler tests of platelet function become available that can potentially be utilized as POC tests or at least within non-specialized laboratories. With the increasing development of new classes of antiplatelet drugs and the known heterogeneity in their biological effects between patients, it may become useful to monitor an individual's response to antiplatelet therapy so that either the dosage and/or the type of drug(s) administered can be titrated or optimized within individual patients to help control and minimize the risk of either thrombosis or bleeding.

The antiplatelet drug aspirin has traditionally been administered at a standard dose with no monitoring of effect, on the assumption that usual doses are two to three times that thought to be required to inhibit allcyclooxygenase-1 (COX-1) activity. However, the lack of a simple, convenient, reliable and clinically relevant test of platelet function has meant that lack of effect in individual patients has gone undetected. With the availability of other classes of antiplatelet drugs (e.g. thienopyridines, new $P2Y_{12}$ antagonists and GPIIb-IIIa antagonists) there is now much interest in the potential utility of platelet function tests to monitor the efficacy of platelet inhibition. The development of GPIIb-IIIa antagonists in particular resulted in the development of a number of new assays to monitor a patient's response (e.g. VerifyNow® IIb/IIIa, flow cytometry of GPIIb-IIIa occupancy), mainly because of their narrow therapeutic window with associated increased risk of bleeding. This, coupled with the now well-studied but poorly-defined phenomenon of "drug resistance" (i.e. the failure of a given antiplatelet drug or treatment to prevent an arterial thrombotic event), has led to an explosion of interest, research and availability of a variety of tests that can potentially monitor an individual's response to antiplatelet therapy.[75] The question remains as to whether these tests are clinically useful, either to predict bleeding or thrombosis. Patient non-compliance to their therapy is also an important but relatively common confounding problem in many studies.[75]

It is well known that there is considerable variation in the response of individuals (either patients or normal controls) to aspirin, clopidogrel and GPIIb-IIIa antagonists as measured by various platelet function tests. Those individuals who respond poorly to a given drug are therefore termed "resistant." However, this is a poorly-defined phenomenon and a precise definition of resistance should only relate to the action of a specific drug to inhibit its biochemical target.[76] Many platelet function tests are non-specific (e.g. the PFA-100®) and they do not do this. Resistance may simply represent natural biological variation in a given drug response or may be due to specific or more complicated mechanisms.[77] Is resistance specific to an individual class of drug and related to its mechanism of action, or are there common inherited and/or acquired mechanism(s) that may influence an individual's response to not just one but potentially all antiplatelet drugs?[77] Whatever the mechanism(s), the key question is whether any laboratory tests which detect either resistance or non-response predict clinical events. Until these links are firmly proven within large trials then resistance in the laboratory cannot necessarily be ascribed as a cause of thrombosis. Therefore, except in research trials, it is still not yet clinically useful to test for resistance and change a patient's therapy on the basis of a laboratory test.[75,77,78] The following sections discuss the specific laboratory tests for the three main current choices of antiplatelet drug.

Monitoring aspirin

Aspirin irreversibly inhibits COX-1 resulting in the inhibition of thromboxane (TX) A_2 generation for the entire lifespan of the platelet.[79] Aspirin is an effective antiplatelet agent because it reduces the relative risk of major vascular events and vascular death by about 25% after ischemic stroke and acute coronary syndrome.[80] Regular low doses of aspirin (e.g. 81 mg/day) will result in $> 95\%$ inhibition of thromboxane generation, as shown by arachidonic acid-induced platelet LTA. Therapeutic monitoring was therefore thought to be unnecessary. However, the antiplatelet properties of aspirin have been shown to vary between individuals and recurrent events in some patients could be due to "aspirin resistance" or aspirin non-responsiveness.[76,77] The reported incidence of aspirin non-responsiveness varies widely (between 5%–60%), partly because there is no accepted standard definition based upon either clinical or laboratory criteria. There are also many possible mechanisms for aspirin resistance which have been discussed in detail elsewhere.[77,81] Recently it has been proposed that the term "aspirin resistance" should only be utilized as a description of the failure of aspirin to inhibit TXA_2 production, irrespective of a non-specific test of platelet function.[76] This is because there are many other biochemical pathways that can potentially bypass COX-1 even if this enzyme is inhibited. Depending upon the test system employed, "aspirin resistance" or more correctly an aspirin non-responsiveness may therefore be detected even if COX-1 is fully blocked.[76] Recent studies also suggest that, in compliant patients, the incidence of aspirin resistance is rare using methods dependent on COX-1 activity.[66,82] Addition of *in vitro* aspirin to samples followed by retesting should also be an important consideration for testing compliance.[83]

Many tests have been used to assess the influence of aspirin on platelets and aspirin resistance, including arachidonic acid- and ADP-induced LTA, ADP- and collagen-induced impedance aggregation, VerifyNow® Aspirin, PFA-100®, Thromboelastography® (TEG — Platelet Mapping System®), flow cytometry using arachidonic acid stimulation and serum and urinary thromboxane.[75] Tests should ideally be performed pre- and post-drug. Some of the tests have been claimed to be predictive of adverse clinical events.[75] However, the large majority of these studies are small and often statistically underpowered to completely answer whether each test can reliably predict the small number of adverse outcomes that were observed in each study.[77,81]

Although preliminary results from some studies could suggest that responses to aspirin should be monitored, there are additional problems in that LTA is time-consuming, difficult and cannot realistically be performed on large numbers of patients in routine practice. However, the simpler tests of platelet function (e.g. PFA-100®, VerifyNow® Aspirin, TEG Platelet Mapping® and urinary thromboxane) could offer the possibility of rapid and reliable identification of aspirin non-responsive patients, without the requirement of a specialized laboratory. The PFA-100® usually gives a prolongation in the Collagen/Epinephrine (CEPI) CT in response to aspirin, with the Collagen/ADP (CADP) CT usually remaining within the normal range.[84,85] A number of studies have observed that an appreciable number of both normals and patients are "aspirin resistant" or fail to respond in terms of prolongation of their CEPI CT in response to aspirin.[86–93] Because the PFA-100® is a global high-shear test of platelet function, many variables have been shown to influence the CT including VWF levels, platelet count and hematocrit.[52] In patients identified with "aspirin resistance" by the PFA-100®, a number of studies have shown that VWF levels are elevated in non-responders when compared to responders.[91,92,94] As the CEPI CT is highly dependent upon VWF and other variables, pre- and post-aspirin CTs should ideally be determined, because the true aspirin response may be masked by either short or prolonged CTs before the drug is given.[76] Also CADP CTs are lower in these patients, which may be caused by a combination of high VWF but also increased sensitivity to collagen and ADP as shown by LTA.[91,95,96] It is therefore possible that the apparent increased sensitivity of the PFA-100® to detecting an aspirin non-responsiveness is caused by a combination of these factors, resulting in the normalization of the CT despite adequate COX-1 blockade by aspirin. It is therefore not surprising that the incidence of aspirin non-responders is reportedly much higher with the PFA-100® than other tests.[97,98] It is likely that the PFA-100® is detecting not only resistance (i.e. failure to inhibit COX-1) but also individuals who are able to give normal CEPI CTs despite adequate COX-1 blockade. The question remains whether or not either of these groups of patients are at increased risk of thrombosis. Preliminary data suggests that PFA-100® CEPI CTs were non-informative in patients with stable coronary artery disease, in contrast to LTA.[99–102] However, another study suggests that the PFA-100® could be informative,[103] and that shortened CTs with the CADP cartridge (which is not affected by aspirin) may also be predictive.[95,104–106] Further large prospective studies on the PFA-100® are required.

The VerifyNow® Aspirin assay provides a true POC test for monitoring responses to aspirin. The test offers the possibility of rapid and reliable identification of aspirin resistance or non-responsiveness without the requirement of a specialized laboratory or LTA. Indeed, the test has United States

Food and Drug Administration (FDA) approval for monitoring aspirin therapy and is being used by some cardiologists and general practitioners in the US. The original VerifyNow® Aspirin cartridge contains fibrinogen-coated beads and a platelet activator (metallic cations and propyl gallate) to stimulate the COX-1 pathway and activate platelets.[107] Ideally, the test should produce similar results to those obtained by arachidonic acid-induced LTA. One study showed an 87% agreement with epinephrine-induced LTA.[108] Previous data comparing propyl gallate and other agonists by platelet aggregometry suggest that this agonist detects a lower number of responders in volunteers receiving either 100 or 400 mg of aspirin.[107] A more recent study compared LTA with VerifyNow® Aspirin and PFA-100® in 100 stroke patients on low-dose aspirin therapy and demonstrated that aspirin non-responsiveness was not only higher in both POC tests, but that agreement between the tests was poor and few patients were non-responsive by all three tests.[97] Nevertheless, the VerifyNow® Aspirin test can potentially identify a correlation between aspirin non-responders, adverse clinical outcomes and aspirin dose.[109–112] Since the end of 2004, the VerifyNow® Aspirin cartridge has been modified and arachidonic acid has replaced propyl gallate as the principle agonist. Further studies are therefore warranted to relate adverse clinical outcomes to the new VerifyNow® Aspirin assay and to see whether changing therapy based upon the result can also improve outcomes.

Because aspirin inhibits COX-1, measurement of TXA_2 and its metabolites either within serum or urine provides a potentially relatively simple way to monitor aspirin therapy. *In vivo*, TXA_2 is rapidly converted into the more stable and inert metabolite TXB_2 which is further metabolized to 11-dehydro TXB_2, the major product found in urine. Measurement of TXB_2 by various immunoassays can facilitate an indirect assessment of the capacity of platelets to form TXA_2. Assays can be standardized so that TXB_2 is measured either within serum derived from whole blood clotted for 30 minutes at 37°C or in supernatants derived from PRP or purified platelets (with standardized platelet counts) activated by agonists to stimulate COX-1 activity. The metabolite 11-dehydro TXB_2 can also be measured within urine samples and the assay is also commercially available as the AspirinWorks® test. This assay has the advantage that it is non-invasive and one large study suggested that high levels of urinary 11-dehydro TXB_2 are associated with adverse clinical events in patients receiving low dose aspirin.[113]

Monitoring clopidogrel

Clopidogrel (Plavix) is a prodrug that is metabolized by cytochrome P450 in the liver to an active metabolite that specifically and irreversibly blocks the platelet ADP $P2Y_{12}$ receptor.[114] Platelet inhibition by clopidogrel is both dose- and time-dependent and patients are usually given a loading dose of 300–600 mg and then maintained on 75 mg/day. The CAPRIE trial showed that clopidogrel prevented more thrombotic vascular events than aspirin (RRR 8.7%) in patients with known atherosclerosis.[115] The CURE trial showed aspirin plus clopidogrel was 20% more effective than aspirin alone in acute coronary syndromes,[116] but the MATCH study showed equivalence of aspirin plus clopidogrel with clopidogrel alone in patients with ischemic stroke or transient ischemic attack (TIA).[117] Combination therapy is regarded as the gold standard during percutaneous coronary intervention (PCI).[118] However, inter-individual variability in platelet response to clopidogrel has been observed,[119] and 5%–10% of patients still experience acute or subacute thrombosis after coronary stent implantation.[76,120–122] The phenomenon of "clopidogrel resistance" has been estimated to be between 4% and 30%. The definition of clopidogrel resistance is even more complex than aspirin resistance because the physiological degree of inhibition detected by ADP-induced LTA can vary widely between individuals, especially as ADP can also activate platelets via a second receptor, $P2Y_1$, and there is inter-individual variability of cytochrome P450 activity.[114] There is an inverse correlation between P450 3A4 activity and platelet aggregation, and other drugs can either promote or inhibit metabolism to a certain degree.[123] Pre-existing variability in ADP responsiveness is also an important variable and may provide an explanation for response variability (Fig. 5).[124] Many mechanisms of clopidogrel resistance have also been proposed, some of which are similar to aspirin.[75]

Laboratory responses to clopidogrel and other $P2Y_{12}$ inhibitors are largely based upon monitoring ADP-stimulated responses.[125] Platelets are stimulated with ADP and responses are monitored using either LTA, the VerifyNow® P2Y12 assay, TEG Platelet Mapping System® or flow cytometric analysis of activation-dependent markers (e.g. P-selectin, PAC-1), flow cytometric analysis of intracellular signaling by monitoring vasodilator-stimulated phosphoprotein (VASP) or Plateletworks®.[26,30,114,125] Ideally, responses are monitored pre- and post-drug, although this is not always

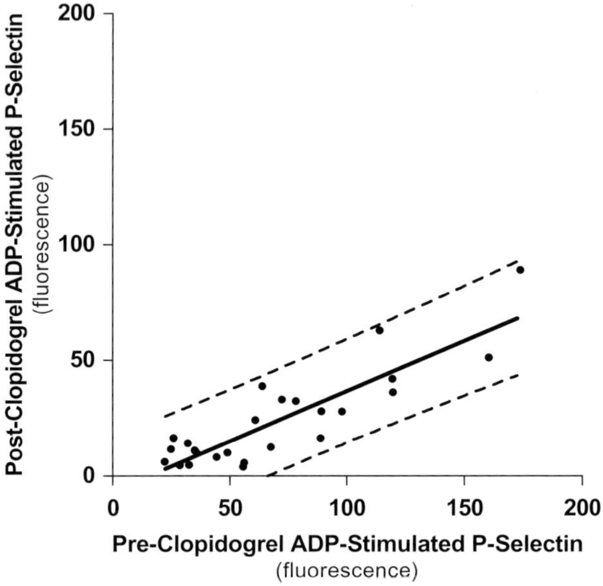

Fig. 5. Pre-clopidogrel response to ADP predicts post-clopidogrel response to ADP in non-aspirin-treated healthy subjects. Before and five hours after oral administration of 300 mg clopidogrel to healthy volunteers, anticoagulated diluted whole blood was stimulated *ex vivo* with 20 μM ADP. Platelet surface P-selectin was determined by whole blood flow cytometry. Dashed lines represent 95% prediction band of the regression line. Pearson $r = 0.8703$, $p < 0.0001$, $n = 25$ subjects. Reprinted with permission from Blackwell Publishing Ltd.[124]

possible in the clinical world. LTA using 5 or 20 μM ADP can be used to arbitrarily classify patients into three categories: non-responders, intermediate responders and responders, based upon measuring the change in (delta) aggregation at baseline and post-drug.[126] Non-responders can be defined with a delta aggregation of < 10%. Studies have shown that there is considerable variation in patient response to clopidogrel and up to 30% of patients may be non-responders. The largest analysis so far has found 4% of 544 patients to be hypo-responsive to clopidogrel.[119] More recent data suggests that a proportion of patients are probably under-dosed and that a 600 mg loading dose significantly reduces the number of non-responders when compared to 300 mg.[126–128] There is still the critical unresolved question as to whether *in vitro* lack of responsiveness to clopidogrel correlates with an increased incidence of adverse events.

ADP-induced LTA is probably not very practical to test on large numbers of clinical samples outside a research setting. Also, as residual $P2Y_1$ function can potentially widely vary despite $P2Y_{12}$ inhibition, this could not only explain some of the heterogeneity observed with LTA but suggests that ADP alone may not be specific enough to measure the effect of clopidogrel and other $P2Y_{12}$ antagonists.[129] Despite these problems, Matetzsky *et al.* found, in a small study, evidence that ADP-induced LTA predicted adverse events and that this assay also correlated with epinephrine-induced LTA and the cone and plate(let) analyzer.[130] The VerifyNow instrument was originally designed to overcome the major limitations of LTA and can be used as a POC test. The VerifyNow® P2Y12 cartridge has become available for monitoring clopidogrel and other $P2Y_{12}$ antagonists. The assay uses prostaglandin (PG) E_1 in addition to ADP to increase intracellular cyclic adenosine monophosphate (cAMP), theoretically enhancing the sensitivity and specificity of the test for ADP-induced activation of platelets via $P2Y_{12}$.[131,132] The PGE_1 should suppress the activation of platelets by $P2Y_1$. The VERITAS (The Verify Thrombosis Risk Assessment) trial will determine if the VerifyNow® P2Y12 test is a reliable and sensitive measure for monitoring clopidogrel therapy, although the exact cut-off in this assay remains to be defined.

The combination of ADP and PGE_1 is also used in the flow cytometric-based VASP assay (BioCytex, Marseilles, France)[129,133] The principle of this assay is to measure the phosphorylation of VASP, which is theoretically proportional to the level of inhibition of the $P2Y_{12}$ receptor. Comparison of the VASP assay with LTA shows that the level of inhibition is higher in the flow cytometry assay, because non-specific aggregation can occur via ADP stimulation of $P2Y_1$ during aggregation.[129] Recent data indeed show that the phosphorylation of VASP correlates with inhibition of LTA but not platelet surface expression of P-selectin or the PFA-100® CT.[125] The latter test, with which variable results have been observed, is considered unsuitable for monitoring clopidogrel.[52,134–136] Theoretically the PFA-100® CADP cartridge may be more suitable for monitoring $P2Y_{12}$ antagonists than the CEPI cartridge, but both collagen activation and ADP acting through the $P2Y_1$ receptor, along with the high shear conditions, may be normally sufficient to largely overcome $P2Y_{12}$ blockade.[114] There may be also be a degree of time- and dose-dependence. It has also been observed that there is synergy with clopidogrel/aspirin combination therapy, demonstrated as prolongation of both CADP and CEPI CTs.[137,138]

Assessment of platelet function by a variety of tests in correlation with clinical outcomes will also be necessary to define responsiveness to clopidogrel and other P2Y12 antagonists. Preliminary data from the CREST (Clopidogrel Resistance and Stent Thrombosis) study by Gurbel *et al.* show differences between VASP, LTA and activated GPIIb-IIIa responsiveness to ADP between patients with and without subacute stent thrombosis (SAT).[139] Comparing data from patients with ($n = 20$) and without SAT ($n = 100$) suggests that clopidogrel response variability to ADP is significantly associated with an increased risk of SAT.[139] This, coupled with other studies on post-discharge and post-PCI events, suggests that high post-treatment *ex vivo* reactivity to ADP may indeed be an important risk factor for adverse clinical events.[130,133,140]

Carefully controlled, large randomized trials will be required to define an inadequate response to $P2Y_{12}$ inhibition for an individual test and to show that this correlates with adverse clinical events. Without such data, therapy should not be altered based upon the results of any of the tests that purport to determine responsiveness to a $P2Y_{12}$ antagonist. The new RESISTOR (Research Evaluation to Study Individuals who Show Thromboxane or $P2Y_{12}$ Resistance) trial that is currently underway in 600 PCI patients may determine if the level of $P2Y_{12}$ inhibition correlates with clinical outcome and if changing therapy in resistant patients improves outcome.

The development and clinical application of thienopyridines such as clopidogrel has proven that the $P2Y_{12}$ inhibitor is an attractive target for the development of new drugs. As thienopyridines are metabolized to their active derivatives by the liver, a number of direct antagonists have also been developed (e.g. cangrelor and AZD6140).[114] Some new thienopyridines (e.g. prasugrel) have also been developed which exhibit superior properties (e.g. higher efficacy, faster onset and longer duration of action) over clopidogrel.[114] As some of the observed inter-individual heterogeneity of clopidogrel responsiveness may be caused by differences in liver metabolism, it will be interesting to determine whether the incidence of non-responsiveness is lower or even eradicated with these new drugs and whether high post-treatment reactivity to ADP remains a potential significant problem.

Monitoring GPIIb-IIIa antagonists

The identification of the importance of the GPIIb-IIIa complex (integrin αIIbβ3) in mediating platelet aggregation (i.e. the final common pathway of platelet activation) suggested that this receptor would be another attractive target for antithrombotic therapy. The platelet GPIIb-IIIa antagonists (abciximab, tirofiban and eptifibatide) have now become an important class of antiplatelet agents that are widely used for the prevention of thrombotic complications in patients undergoing PCI or presenting with acute coronary syndromes. Early observations on the inhibition of thrombus formation within animal models not only established a strong correlation between the level of GPIIb-IIIa blockade and the prevention of thrombus formation but demonstrated steep dose-response curves.[141,142] It became rapidly apparent that a certain level of GPIIb-IIIa inhibition was required for the optimal efficacy of GPIIb-IIIa antagonists. This strongly suggested that monitoring of platelet inhibition could be important in patients treated with these agents. Monitoring GPIIb-IIIa antagonists can be performed by a variety of tests including LTA, WBA, flow cytometry, and radiolabeled antibody binding assays.[143] However some of these tests are time-consuming, expensive and are usually performed within specialized laboratories. Given the widespread clinical use of these GPIIb-IIIa antagonists in cardiology, there existed a demand for a simple, inexpensive and rapid method that could be utilized as a POC test either at the bedside or in the clinic, so that the degree of GPIIb-IIIa blockade could be also be potentially determined by non-specialists. The VerifyNow® system was originally developed to meet this demand. The assay principle was developed based upon experiments using fibrinogen-coated beads and TRAP which facilitated the rapid visual analysis of the degree of GPIIb-IIIa blockade.[21] The basis of the VerifyNow® IIb/IIIa assay is that fibrinogen-coated beads will agglutinate in whole blood in direct proportion to the degree of platelet activation and GPIIb-IIIa exposure.[19] The presence of a GPIIb-IIIa antagonist will therefore decrease the amount of agglutination in proportion to the level of inhibition achieved.

Initial *in vitro* evaluations of the VerifyNow® IIb/IIIa assay demonstrated good correlations with either LTA in PRP or radiolabeled receptor binding assays.[19] Studies in patients receiving either abciximab or other GPIIb-IIIa antagonists also demonstrated good correlations with LTA.[144,145]

A slightly modified Plateletworks® POC assay was recently reported to correlate more strongly than VerifyNow® IIb/IIIa with LTA in measuring platelet inhibition by GPIIb-IIIa antagonists.[27] GOLD (AU — Assessing Ultegra), a large prospective multicenter study, showed a significant association between the level of platelet inhibition by the VerifyNow® IIb/IIIa assay and clinical outcomes.[146] This suggests that the device has clinical utility, although no study has yet been performed to determine whether titration of GPIIb-IIIa therapy based upon the VerifyNow® IIb/IIIa test result decreases adverse events. The PFA-100 has also been utilized to monitor GPIIb-IIIa blockade and correlates well with LTA and receptor occupancy measurements.[147–149] Although many patients give non-closure or > 300 second CT in the PFA-100 following GPIIb-IIIa antagonist treatment, one study suggests that failure to observe non-closure may be associated with an increased risk of cardiac events.[149] This warrants further investigation.

Conclusions

As summarized in this chapter, many tests of platelet function are now available for clinical use, and some of these tests have been shown to predict clinical outcomes after antiplatelet therapy. However, in most of these studies, the number of major adverse clinical events was low, and additional studies are therefore needed. Most importantly, no published studies address the clinical effectiveness of altering therapy based on the results of monitoring antiplatelet therapy. Therefore: (1) the correct treatment, if any, of "resistance" to antiplatelet therapy is unknown and (2) other than in research trials, it is not currently appropriate to monitor antiplatelet therapy in patients or to change therapy based on such tests.[75–77] A clinically meaningful definition of "resistance" to antiplatelet drugs needs to be developed, based on data linking drug-dependent laboratory tests to clinical outcomes in patients.

References

1. George JN. Platelets. *Lancet* 2000;**355**:1531–1539.
2. The British Society for Haematology BCSH Haemostasis and Thrombosis Task Force. Guidelines on platelet function testing. *J Clin Pathol* 1988;**41**:1322–1330.

3. Gawaz M, Langer H, May AE. Platelets in inflammation and atherogenesis. *J Clin Invest* 2005;**115**:3378–3384.
4. Ruggeri ZM. Platelets in atherothrombosis. *Nat Med* 2002;**8**:1227–1234.
5. Harrison P. Platelet function analysis. *Blood Rev* 2005;**19**:111–123.
6. Harrison P. Progress in the assessment of platelet function. *Br J Haematol* 2000;**111**:733–744.
7. de Gaetano G. A new blood corpuscle: an impossible interview with Giulio Bizzozero. *Thromb Haemost* 2001;**86**:973–979.
8. Duke WW. The relation of blood platelets to hemorrhagic disease. Description of a method for determining the bleeding time and the coagulation time and report of three cases of hemorrahagic disease relieved by blood transfusion. *JAMA* 1910;**55**:1185–1192.
9. Harker LA, Slichter SJ. The bleeding time as a screening test for evaluation of platelet function. *N Engl J Med* 1972;**287**:155–159.
10. Nilsson IM, Magnusson S, Borchgrevink C. The Duke and Ivy methods for determination of the bleeding time. *Thromb Diath Haemorrh* 1963;**10**: 223–234.
11. Rodgers RP, Levin J. A critical reappraisal of the bleeding time. *Semin Thromb Hemost* 1990;**16**:1–20.
12. Lind SE. The bleeding time does not predict surgical bleeding. *Blood* 1991;**77**:2547–2552.
13. Peterson P, Hayes TE, Arkin CF, Bovill EG, Fairweather RB, Rock WA, Jr, Triplett DA, Brandt JT. The preoperative bleeding time test lacks clinical benefit: College of American Pathologists' and American Society of Clinical Pathologists' position article. *Arch Surg* 1998;**133**:134–139.
14. Born GV. Aggregation of blood platelets by adenosine diphosphate and its reversal. *Nature* 1962;**194**:927–929.
15. O'Brien JM. Platelet aggregation. II. Some results from a new method of study. *J Clin Pathol* 1962;**15**:452–481.
16. Zhou L, Schmaier AH. Platelet aggregation testing in platelet-rich plasma: description of procedures with the aim to develop standards in the field. *Am J Clin Pathol* 2005;**123**:172–183.
17. Moffat KA, Ledford-Kraemer MR, Nichols WL, Hayward CP. Variability in clinical laboratory practice in testing for disorders of platelet function: results of two surveys of the North American Specialized Coagulation Laboratory Association. *Thromb Haemost* 2005;**93**:549–553.
18. Cardinal DC, Flower RJ. The electronic aggregometer: a novel device for assessing platelet behavior in blood. *J Pharmacol Methods* 1980;**3**: 135–158.

19. Smith JW, Steinhubl SR, Lincoff AM, Coleman JC, Lee TT, Hillman RS, Coller BS. Rapid platelet-function assay: an automated and quantitative cartridge-based method. *Circulation* 1999;**99**:620–625.
20. Kereiakes DJ, Mueller M, Howard W, Lacock P, Anderson LC, Broderick TM, Roth EM, Whang DD, Abbottsmith CW. Efficacy of abciximab induced platelet blockade using a rapid point of care assay. *J Thromb Thrombolysis* 1999;**7**:265–276.
21. Coller BS, Lang D, Scudder LE. Rapid and simple platelet function assay to assess glycoprotein IIb/IIIa receptor blockade. *Circulation* 1997;**95**: 860–867.
22. Fox SC, Burgess-Wilson M, Heptinstall S, Mitchell JR. Platelet aggregation in whole blood determined using the Ultra-Flo 100 Platelet Counter. *Thromb Haemost* 1982;**48**:327–329.
23. Heptinstall S, Fox S, Crawford J, Hawkins M. Inhibition of platelet aggregation in whole blood by dipyridamole and aspirin. *Thromb Res* 1986;**42**: 215–223.
24. Glenn JR, White AE, Johnson A, Fox SC, Behan MW, Dolan G, Heptinstall S. Leukocyte count and leukocyte ecto-nucleotidase are major determinants of the effects of adenosine triphosphate and adenosine diphosphate on platelet aggregation in human blood. *Platelets* 2005;**16**:159–170.
25. Carville DG, Schleckser PA, Guyer KE, Corsello M, Walsh MM. Whole blood platelet function assay on the ICHOR point-of-care hematology analyzer. *J Extra Corpor Technol* 1998;**30**:171–177.
26. Craft RM, Chavez JJ, Snider CC, Muenchen RA, Carroll RC. Comparison of modified Thrombelastograph and Plateletworks whole blood assays to optical platelet aggregation for monitoring reversal of clopidogrel inhibition in elective surgery patients. *J Lab Clin Med* 2005;**145**:309–315.
27. White MM, Krishnan R, Kueter TJ, Jacoski MV, Jennings LK. The use of the point of care Helena ICHOR/Plateletworks and the Accumetrics Ultegra RPFA for assessment of platelet function with GPIIB-IIIa antagonists. *J Thromb Thrombolysis* 2004;**18**:163–169.
28. Lennon MJ, Gibbs NM, Weightman WM, McGuire D, Michalopoulos N. A comparison of Plateletworks and platelet aggregometry for the assessment of aspirin-related platelet dysfunction in cardiac surgical patients. *J Cardiothorac Vasc Anesth* 2004;**18**:136–140.
29. Nicholson NS, Panzer-Knodle SG, Haas NF, Taite BB, Szalony JA, Page JD, Feigen LP, Lansky DM, Salyers AK. Assessment of platelet function assays. *Am Heart J* 1998;**135**:S170–S178.

30. Mobley JE, Bresee SJ, Wortham DC, Craft RM, Snider CC, Carroll RC. Frequency of nonresponse antiplatelet activity of clopidogrel during pre-treatment for cardiac catheterization. *Am J Cardiol* 2004;**93**:456–458.
31. Lakkis NM, George S, Thomas E, Ali M, Guyer K, Carville D. Use of ICHOR-platelet works to assess platelet function in patients treated with GP IIb/IIIa inhibitors. *Catheter Cardiovasc Interv* 2001;**53**:346–351.
32. Wu KK, Hoak JC. A new method for the quantitative detection of platelet aggregates in patients with arterial insufficiency. *Lancet* 1974;**2**:924–926.
33. Grotemeyer KH. The platelet-reactivity-test — a useful "by-product" of the blood-sampling procedure? *Thromb Res* 1991;**61**:423–431.
34. Koscielny J, Meyer O, Kiesewetter H, Jung F, Latza R. Platelet reactivity index by Grotemeyer. *Hamostaseologie* 2004;**24**:207–210.
35. Hellem AJ. The adhesiveness of human blood platelets *in vitro*. *Scand J Clin Lab Invest* 1960;**12**(Suppl):1–117.
36. O'Brien JR, Etherington MD. Anti-glycoprotein Ib causes platelet aggregation: different effects of blocking glycoprotein Ib and glycoprotein IIb/IIIa in the high shear filterometer. *Blood Coagul Fibrinolysis* 1998;**9**:453–461.
37. O'Brien JR, Salmon GP. Shear stress activation of platelet glycoprotein IIb/IIIa plus von Willebrand factor causes aggregation: filter blockage and the long bleeding time in von Willebrand's disease. *Blood* 1987;**70**:1354–1361.
38. Krischek B, Morgenstern E, Mestres P, Klinkhardt U, Brannath W, Wieding U, Nemeh A, Heinrich W, Schenk J, Wenzel T, Wenzel E. Adhesion, spreading, and aggregation of platelets in flowing blood and the reliability of the retention test Homburg. *Semin Thromb Hemost* 2005;**31**:449–457.
39. Krischek B, Brannath W, Klinkhardt U, Graff J, Wieding U, Nemeh A, Heinrich W, Schenk J, Wenzel T, Wenzel E. Role of the retention test homburg in evaluating platelet hyperactivity and in monitoring therapy with antiplatelet drugs. *Semin Thromb Hemost* 2005;**31**:458–463.
40. Nowak G, Wiesenburg A, Schumann A, Bucha E. Platelet adhesion assay — a new quantitative whole blood test to measure platelet function. *Semin Thromb Hemost* 2005;**31**:470–475.
41. Falati S, Gross PL, Merrill-Skoloff G, Sim D, Flaumenhaft R, Celi A, Furie BC, Furie B. *In vivo* models of platelet function and thrombosis: study of real-time thrombus formation. *Methods Mol Biol* 2004;**272**:187–197.
42. Falati S, Gross P, Merrill-Skoloff G, Furie BC, Furie B. Real-time *in vivo* imaging of platelets, tissue factor and fibrin during arterial thrombus formation in the mouse. *Nat Med* 2002;**8**:1175–1181.
43. Furie B, Furie BC. Thrombus formation *in vivo*. *J Clin Invest* 2005;**115**:3355–3362.

44. Gorog DA, Kovacs IB. Thrombotic status analyser. Measurement of platelet-rich thrombus formation and lysis in native blood. *Thromb Haemost* 1995;**73**:514–520.
45. Li CK, Hoffmann TJ, Hsieh PY, Malik S, Watson WC. The Xylum Clot Signature Analyzer: a dynamic flow system that simulates vascular injury. *Thromb Res* 1998;**92**:S67–S77.
46. Fricke W, Kouides P, Kessler C, Schmaier AH, Krijanovski Y, Jagadeesan K, Joist J. A multicenter clinical evaluation of the Clot Signature Analyzer. *J Thromb Haemost* 2004;**2**:763–768.
47. Gorog P, Ahmed A. Haemostatometer: a new *in vitro* technique for assessing haemostatic activity of blood. *Thromb Res* 1984;**34**:341–357.
48. Spectre G, Brill A, Gural A, Shenkman B, Touretsky N, Mosseri E, Savion N, Varon D. A new point-of-care method for monitoring anti-platelet therapy: application of the cone and plate(let) analyzer. *Platelets* 2005;**16**: 293–299.
49. Kenet G, Lubetsky A, Shenkman B, Tamarin I, Dardik R, Rechavi G, Barzilai A, Martinowitz U, Savion N, Varon D. Cone and platelet analyser (CPA): a new test for the prediction of bleeding among thrombocytopenic patients. *Br J Haematol* 1998;**101**:255–259.
50. Varon D, Lashevski I, Brenner B, Beyar R, Lanir N, Tamarin I, Savion N. Cone and plate(let) analyzer: monitoring glycoprotein IIb/IIIa antagonists and von Willebrand disease replacement therapy by testing platelet deposition under flow conditions. *Am Heart J* 1998;**135**:S187–S193.
51. Harrison P. The role of PFA-100 testing in the investigation and management of haemostatic defects in children and adults. *Br J Haematol* 2005;**130**:3–10.
52. Jilma B. Platelet function analyzer (PFA-100): a tool to quantify congenital or acquired platelet dysfunction. *J Lab Clin Med* 2001;**138**:152–163.
53. Kundu SK, Heilmann EJ, Sio R, Garcia C, Ostgaard RA. Characterization of an *in vitro* platelet function analyzer — PFA-100. *Clin Appl Thromb Hemost* 1996;**2**:241–249.
54. Kundu SK, Heilmann EJ, Sio R, Garcia C, Davidson RM, Ostgaard RA. Description of an *in vitro* platelet function analyzer — PFA-100. *Semin Thromb Hemost* 1995;**21**(Suppl 2):106–112.
55. Caen JP, Rosa JP. Platelet-vessel wall interaction: from the bedside to molecules. *Thromb Haemost* 1995;**74**:18–24.
56. Gerotziafas GT, Depasse F, Busson J, Leflem L, Elalamy I, Samama MM. Towards a standardization of thrombin generation assessment: the influence of tissue factor, platelets and phospholipids concentration on the normal values of Thrombogram-Thrombinoscope assay. *Thromb J* 2005;**3**:16.

57. Al DR, Peyvandi F, Santagostino E, Giansily M, Mannucci PM, Schved JF, Beguin S, Hemker HC. The thrombogram in rare inherited coagulation disorders: its relation to clinical bleeding. *Thromb Haemost* 2002;**88**: 576–582.
58. Hemker HC, Beguin S. Thrombin generation in plasma: its assessment via the endogenous thrombin potential. *Thromb Haemost* 1995;**74**:134–138.
59. Coiffic A, Cazes E, Janvier G, Forestier F, Lanza F, Nurden A, Nurden P. Inhibition of platelet aggregation by abciximab but not by aspirin can be detected by a new point-of-care test, the hemostatus. *Thromb Res* 1999;**95**:83–91.
60. Despotis GJ, Levine V, Saleem R, Spitznagel E, Joist JH. Use of point-of-care test in identification of patients who can benefit from desmopressin during cardiac surgery: a randomised controlled trial. *Lancet* 1999;**354**:106–110.
61. Despotis GJ, Levine V, Filos KS, Santoro SA, Joist JH, Spitznagel E, Goodnough LT. Evaluation of a new point-of-care test that measures PAF-mediated acceleration of coagulation in cardiac surgical patients. *Anesthesiology* 1996;**85**:1311–1323.
62. Luddington RJ. Thrombelastography/thromboelastometry. *Clin Lab Haematol* 2005;**27**:81–90.
63. Salooja N, Perry DJ. Thrombelastography. *Blood Coagul Fibrinolysis* 2001;**12**:327–337.
64. Hartert H. Thrombelastography, a method for physical analysis of blood coagulation. *Z Gesamte Exp Med* 1951;**117**:189–203.
65. Lang T, Bauters A, Braun SL, Potzsch B, von Pape KW, Kolde HJ, Lakner M. Multi-centre investigation on reference ranges for ROTEM thromboelastometry. *Blood Coagul Fibrinolysis* 2005;**16**:301–310.
66. Tantry US, Bliden KP, Gurbel PA. Overestimation of platelet aspirin resistance detection by thrombelastograph platelet mapping and validation by conventional aggregometry using arachidonic acid stimulation. *J Am Coll Cardiol* 2005;**46**:1705–1709.
67. Bowbrick VA, Mikhailidis DP, Stansby G. Value of thromboelastography in the assessment of platelet function. *Clin Appl Thromb Hemost* 2003;**9**: 137–142.
68. Carr ME, Jr, Zekert SL. Measurement of platelet-mediated force development during plasma clot formation. *Am J Med Sci* 1991;**302**:13–18.
69. Carr ME, Martin EJ, Kuhn JG, Spiess BD. Onset of force development as a marker of thrombin generation in whole blood: the thrombin generation time (TGT). *J Thromb Haemost* 2003;**1**:1977–1983.
70. Carr ME, Jr. Development of platelet contractile force as a research and clinical measure of platelet function. *Cell Biochem Biophys* 2003;**38**:55–78.

71. Carr ME, Jr. Measurement of platelet force: the Hemodyne hemostasis analyzer. *Clin Lab Manage Rev* 1995;**9**:312–318, 320.
72. Michelson AD, Furman MI. Laboratory markers of platelet activation and their clinical significance. *Curr Opin Hematol* 1999;**6**:342–348.
73. Schmitz G, Rothe G, Ruf A, Barlage S, Tschope D, Clemetson KJ, Goodall AH, Michelson AD, Nurden AT, Shankey TV. European Working Group on Clinical Cell Analysis: Consensus protocol for the flow cytometric characterisation of platelet function. *Thromb Haemost* 1998;**79**:885–896.
74. Michelson AD. Flow cytometry: a clinical test of platelet function. *Blood* 1996;**87**:4925–4936.
75. Michelson AD. Platelet function testing in cardiovascular diseases. *Circulation* 2004;**110**:e489–e493.
76. Cattaneo M. Aspirin and clopidogrel: efficacy, safety, and the issue of drug resistance. *Arterioscler Thromb Vasc Biol* 2004;**24**:1980–1987.
77. Michelson AD, Cattaneo M, Eikelboom JW, Gurbel P, Kottke-Marchant K, Kunicki TJ, Pulcinelli FM, Cerletti C, Rao AK. Aspirin resistance: position paper of the Working Group on Aspirin Resistance. *J Thromb Haemost* 2005;**3**:1309–1311.
78. Szczeklik A, Musial J, Undas A, Sanak M. Aspirin resistance. *J Thromb Haemost* 2005;**3**:1655–1662.
79. Roth GJ, Majerus PW. The mechanism of the effect of aspirin on human platelets. I. Acetylation of a particulate fraction protein. *J Clin Invest* 1975;**56**:624–632.
80. Antithrombotic Trialists' Collaboration. Collaborative meta-analysis of randomised trials of antiplatelet therapy for prevention of death, myocardial infarction, and stroke in high risk patients. *BMJ* 2002;**324**:71–86.
81. Rocca B, Patrono C. Determinants of the interindividual variability in response to antiplatelet drugs. *J Thromb Haemost* 2005;**3**:1597–1602.
82. Schwartz KA, Schwartz DE, Ghosheh K, Reeves MJ, Barber K, DeFranco A. Compliance as a critical consideration in patients who appear to be resistant to aspirin after healing of myocardial infarction. *Am J Cardiol* 2005;**95**:973–975.
83. Weber AA, Przytulski B, Schanz A, Hohlfeld T, Schror K. Towards a definition of aspirin resistance: a typological approach. *Platelets* 2002;**13**:37–40.
84. Homoncik M, Jilma B, Hergovich N, Stohlawetz P, Panzer S, Speiser W. Monitoring of aspirin (ASA) pharmacodynamics with the platelet function analyzer PFA-100. *Thromb Haemost* 2000;**83**:316–321.
85. Feuring M, Schultz A, Losel R, Wehling M. Monitoring acetylsalicylic acid effects with the platelet function analyzer PFA-100. *Semin Thromb Hemost* 2005;**31**:411–415.

86. Andersen K, Hurlen M, Arnesen H, Seljeflot I. Aspirin non-responsiveness as measured by PFA-100 in patients with coronary artery disease. *Thromb Res* 2002;**108**:37–42.
87. Sambola A, Heras M, Escolar G, Lozano M, Pino M, Martorell T, Torra M, Sanz G. The PFA-100 detects sub-optimal antiplatelet responses in patients on aspirin. *Platelets* 2004;**15**:439–446.
88. Coakley M, Self R, Marchant W, Mackie I, Mallett SV, Mythen M. Use of the platelet function analyser (PFA-100) to quantify the effect of low dose aspirin in patients with ischaemic heart disease. *Anaesthesia* 2005;**60**:1173–1178.
89. Coma-Canella I, Velasco A, Castano S. Prevalence of aspirin resistance measured by PFA-100. *Int J Cardiol* 2005;**101**:71–76.
90. Peters AJ, Borries M, Gradaus F, Jax TW, Schoebel FC, Strauer BE. *In vitro* bleeding test with PFA-100-aspects of controlling individual acetylsalicylic acid induced platelet inhibition in patients with cardiovascular disease. *J Thromb Thrombolysis* 2001;**12**:263–272.
91. Harrison P, Mackie I, Mathur A, Robinson MS, Hong Y, Erusalimsky JD, Machin SJ, Martin JF. Platelet hyper-function in acute coronary syndromes. *Blood Coagul Fibrinolysis* 2005;**16**:557–562.
92. McCabe DJ, Harrison P, Mackie IJ, Sidhu PS, Lawrie AS, Purdy G, Machin SJ, Brown MM. Assessment of the antiplatelet effects of low to medium dose aspirin in the early and late phases after ischaemic stroke and TIA. *Platelets* 2005;**16**:269–280.
93. Alberts MJ, Bergman DL, Molner E, Jovanovic BD, Ushiwata I, Teruya J. Antiplatelet effect of aspirin in patients with cerebrovascular disease. *Stroke* 2004;**35**:175–178.
94. Chakroun T, Gerotziafas G, Robert F, Lecrubier C, Samama MM, Hatmi M, Elalamy I. *In vitro* aspirin resistance detected by PFA-100 closure time: pivotal role of plasma von Willebrand factor. *Br J Haematol* 2004;**124**: 80–85.
95. Frossard M, Fuchs I, Leitner JM, Hsieh K, Vlcek M, Losert H, Domanovits H, Schreiber W, Laggner AN, Jilma B. Platelet function predicts myocardial damage in patients with acute myocardial infarction. *Circulation* 2004;**110**:1392–1397.
96. Macchi L, Christiaens L, Brabant S, Sorel N, Allal J, Mauco G, Brizard A. Resistance to aspirin *in vitro* is associated with increased platelet sensitivity to adenosine diphosphate. *Thromb Res* 2002;**107**:45–49.
97. Harrison P, Segal H, Blasbery K, Furtado C, Silver L, Rothwell PM. Screening for aspirin responsiveness after transient ischemic attack and stroke: comparison of 2 point-of-care platelet function tests with optical aggregometry. *Stroke* 2005;**36**:1001–1005.

98. Gum PA, Kottke-Marchant K, Poggio ED, Gurm H, Welsh PA, Brooks L, Sapp SK, Topol EJ. Profile and prevalence of aspirin resistance in patients with cardiovascular disease. *Am J Cardiol* 2001;**88**:230–235.
99. Gum PA, Kottke-Marchant K, Welsh PA, White J, Topol EJ. A prospective, blinded determination of the natural history of aspirin resistance among stable patients with cardiovascular disease. *J Am Coll Cardiol* 2003;**41**:961–965.
100. Steinhubl SR, Varanasi JS, Goldberg L. Determination of the natural history of aspirin resistance among stable patients with cardiovascular disease. *J Am Coll Cardiol* 2003;**42**:1336–1337.
101. Jilma B. Therapeutic failure or resistance to aspirin. *J Am Coll Cardiol* 2004;**43**:1332–1333.
102. Eikelboom JW, Hankey GJ. Aspirin resistance: a new independent predictor of vascular events? *J Am Coll Cardiol* 2003;**41**:966–968.
103. Grundmann K, Jaschonek K, Kleine B, Dichgans J, Topka H. Aspirin non-responder status in patients with recurrent cerebral ischemic attacks. *J Neurol* 2003;**250**:63–66.
104. Lanza GA, Sestito A, Iacovella S, Morlacchi L, Romagnoli E, Schiavoni G, Crea F, Maseri A, Andreotti F. Relation between platelet response to exercise and coronary angiographic findings in patients with effort angina. *Circulation* 2003;**107**:1378–1382.
105. Fuchs I, Frossard M, Spiel A, Mayr FB, Laggner AN, Jilma B. Platelet hyperfunction and low response to aspirin predict re-events in patients with acute coronary syndromes during long term follow up. *J Thromb Haemost* 2005;**3**(Suppl 1):2142 (abstract).
106. Christie DJ, Kottke-Marchant K, Gorman R. High shear platelet function is associated with major adverse events in patients with stable cardiovascular disease (CVD) despite aspirin therapy. *J. Thrombosis Haemostasis* 2005;**3**(Suppl. 1):2204 (abstract).
107. Stejskal D, Proskova J, Petrzelova A, Bartek J, Oral I, Lacnak B, Horalik D, Sekaninova S. Application of cationic propyl gallate as inducer of thrombocyte aggregation for evaluation of effectiveness of antiaggregation therapy. *Biomed Pap Med Fac Univ Palacky Olomouc Czech Repub* 2001;**145**:69–74.
108. Malinin A, Spergling M, Muhlestein B, Steinhubl S, Serebruany V. Assessing aspirin responsiveness in subjects with multiple risk factors for vascular disease with a rapid platelet function analyzer. *Blood Coagul Fibrinolysis* 2004;**15**:295–301.
109. Wang JC, Ucoin-Barry D, Manuelian D, Monbouquette R, Reisman M, Gray W, Block PC, Block EH, Ladenheim M, Simon DI. Incidence of aspirin nonresponsiveness using the Ultegra Rapid Platelet Function Assay-ASA. *Am J Cardiol* 2003;**92**:1492–1494.

110. Chen WH, Lee PY, Ng W, Kwok JY, Cheng X, Lee SW, Tse HF, Lau CP. Relation of aspirin resistance to coronary flow reserve in patients undergoing elective percutaneous coronary intervention. *Am J Cardiol* 2005;**96**:760–763.
111. Chen WH, Lee PY, Ng W, Tse HF, Lau CP. Aspirin resistance is associated with a high incidence of myonecrosis after non-urgent percutaneous coronary intervention despite clopidogrel pretreatment. *J Am Coll Cardiol* 2004;**43**:1122–1126.
112. Lee PY, Chen WH, Ng W, Cheng X, Kwok JY, Tse HF, Lau CP. Low-dose aspirin increases aspirin resistance in patients with coronary artery disease. *Am J Med* 2005;**118**:723–727.
113. Eikelboom JW, Hirsh J, Weitz JI, Johnston M, Yi Q, Yusuf S. Aspirin-resistant thromboxane biosynthesis and the risk of myocardial infarction, stroke, or cardiovascular death in patients at high risk for cardiovascular events. *Circulation* 2002;**105**:1650–1655.
114. Gachet C. Regulation of platelet functions by P2 receptors. *Annu Rev Pharmacol Toxicol* 2006;**46**:277–300.
115. CAPRIE Steering Committee. A randomised, blinded, trial of clopidogrel versus aspirin in patients at risk of ischaemic events (CAPRIE). *Lancet* 1996;**348**:1329–1339.
116. Mehta SR, Yusuf S, Peters RJ, Bertrand ME, Lewis BS, Natarajan MK, Malmberg K, Rupprecht H, Zhao F, Chrolavicius S, Copland I, Fox KA. Effects of pretreatment with clopidogrel and aspirin followed by long-term therapy in patients undergoing percutaneous coronary intervention: the PCI-CURE study. *Lancet* 2001;**358**:527–533.
117. Diener HC, Bogousslavsky J, Brass LM, Cimminiello C, Csiba L, Kaste M, Leys D, Matias-Guiu J, Rupprecht HJ. Aspirin and clopidogrel compared with clopidogrel alone after recent ischaemic stroke or transient ischaemic attack in high-risk patients (MATCH): randomised, double-blind, placebo-controlled trial. *Lancet* 2004;**364**:331–337.
118. Savi P, Herbert JM. Clopidogrel and ticlopidine: P2Y12 adenosine diphosphate-receptor antagonists for the prevention of atherothrombosis. *Semin Thromb Hemost* 2005;**31**:174–183.
119. Serebruany VL, Steinhubl SR, Berger PB, Malinin AI, Bhatt DL, Topol EJ. Variability in platelet responsiveness to clopidogrel among 544 individuals. *J Am Coll Cardiol* 2005;**45**:246–251.
120. Nguyen TA, Diodati JG, Pharand C. Resistance to clopidogrel: a review of the evidence. *J Am Coll Cardiol* 2005;**45**:1157–1164.
121. Gurbel PA, Bliden KP, Hiatt BL, O'Connor CM. Clopidogrel for coronary stenting: response variability, drug resistance, and the effect of pretreatment platelet reactivity. *Circulation* 2003;**107**:2908–2913.

122. Jaremo P, Lindahl TL, Fransson SG, Richter A. Individual variations of platelet inhibition after loading doses of clopidogrel. *J Intern Med* 2002;**252**:233–238.
123. Lau WC, Gurbel PA, Watkins PB, Neer CJ, Hopp AS, Carville DG, Guyer KE, Tait AR, Bates ER. Contribution of hepatic cytochrome P450 3A4 metabolic activity to the phenomenon of clopidogrel resistance. *Circulation* 2004;**109**:166–171.
124. Michelson AD, Linden MD, Furman MI, Li Y, Barnard MR, Fox ML, Lau WC, McLaughlin TJ, Frelinger AL. Evidence that pre-existent variability in platelet response to ADP accounts for 'clopidogrel resistance'. *J Thromb Haemost* 2007;**5**:75–81.
125. Geiger J, Teichmann L, Grossmann R, Aktas B, Steigerwald U, Walter U, Schinzel R. Monitoring of clopidogrel action: comparison of methods. *Clin Chem* 2005;**51**:957–965.
126. Gurbel PA, Bliden KP, Hayes KM, Yoho JA, Herzog WR, Tantry US. The relation of dosing to clopidogrel responsiveness and the incidence of high post-treatment platelet aggregation in patients undergoing coronary stenting. *J Am Coll Cardiol* 2005;**45**:1392–1396.
127. Muller I, Seyfarth M, Rudiger S, Wolf B, Pogatsa-Murray G, Schomig A, Gawaz M. Effect of a high loading dose of clopidogrel on platelet function in patients undergoing coronary stent placement. *Heart* 2001;**85**:92–93.
128. Gurbel PA, Bliden KP, Zaman KA, Yoho JA, Hayes KM, Tantry US. Clopidogrel loading with eptifibatide to arrest the reactivity of platelets: results of the Clopidogrel Loading With Eptifibatide to Arrest the Reactivity of Platelets (CLEAR PLATELETS) study. *Circulation* 2005;**111**:1153–1159.
129. Aleil B, Ravanat C, Cazenave JP, Rochoux G, Heitz A, Gachet C. Flow cytometric analysis of intraplatelet VASP phosphorylation for the detection of clopidogrel resistance in patients with ischemic cardiovascular diseases. *J Thromb Haemost* 2005;**3**:85–92.
130. Matetzky S, Shenkman B, Guetta V, Shechter M, Bienart R, Goldenberg I, Novikov I, Pres H, Savion N, Varon D, Hod H. Clopidogrel resistance is associated with increased risk of recurrent atherothrombotic events in patients with acute myocardial infarction. *Circulation* 2004;**109**:3171–3175.
131. Fox SC, Behan MW, Heptinstall S. Inhibition of ADP-induced intracellular Ca2+ responses and platelet aggregation by the P2Y12 receptor antagonists AR-C69931MX and clopidogrel is enhanced by prostaglandin E1. *Cell Calcium* 2004;**35**:39–46.
132. Gachet C, Cazenave JP, Ohlmann P, Bouloux C, Defreyn G, Driot F, Maffrand JP. The thienopyridine ticlopidine selectively prevents the

inhibitory effects of ADP but not of adrenaline on cAMP levels raised by stimulation of the adenylate cyclase of human platelets by PGE1. *Biochem Pharmacol* 1990;**40**:2683–2687.

133. Barragan P, Bouvier JL, Roquebert PO, Macaluso G, Commeau P, Comet B, Lafont A, Camoin L, Walter U, Eigenthaler M. Resistance to thienopyridines: clinical detection of coronary stent thrombosis by monitoring of vasodilator-stimulated phosphoprotein phosphorylation. *Catheter Cardiovasc Interv* 2003;**59**:295–302.
134. Golanski J, Pluta J, Baraniak J, Watala C. Limited usefulness of the PFA-100 for the monitoring of ADP receptor antagonists — *in vitro* experience. *Clin Chem Lab Med* 2004;**42**:25–29.
135. Mueller T, Haltmayer M, Poelz W, Haidinger D. Monitoring aspirin 100 mg and clopidogrel 75 mg therapy with the PFA-100 device in patients with peripheral arterial disease. *Vasc Endovasc Surg* 2003;**37**:117–123.
136. Ziegler S, Maca T, Alt E, Speiser W, Schneider B, Minar E. Monitoring of antiplatelet therapy with the PFA-100 in peripheral angioplasty patients. *Platelets* 2002;**13**:493–497.
137. Raman S, Jilma B. Time lag in platelet function inhibition by clopidogrel in stroke patients as measured by PFA-100. *J Thromb Haemost* 2004;**2**:2278–2279.
138. Jilma B. Synergistic antiplatelet effects of clopidogrel and aspirin detected with the PFA-100 in stroke patients. *Stroke* 2003;**34**:849–854.
139. Gurbel PA, Bliden KP, Samara W, Yoho JA, Hayes K, Fissha MZ, Tantry US. Clopidogrel effect on platelet reactivity in patients with stent thrombosis: results of the CREST Study. *J Am Coll Cardiol* 2005;**46**:1827–1832.
140. Muller I, Besta F, Schulz C, Massberg S, Schomig A, Gawaz M. Prevalence of clopidogrel non-responders among patients with stable angina pectoris scheduled for elective coronary stent placement. *Thromb Haemost* 2003;**89**:783–787.
141. Coller BS, Folts JD, Smith SR, Scudder LE, Jordan R. Abolition of *in vivo* platelet thrombus formation in primates with monoclonal antibodies to the platelet GPIIb/IIIa receptor. Correlation with bleeding time, platelet aggregation, and blockade of GPIIb/IIIa receptors. *Circulation* 1989;**80**:1766–1774.
142. Gold HK, Coller BS, Yasuda T, Saito T, Fallon JT, Guerrero JL, Leinbach RC, Ziskind AA, Collen D. Rapid and sustained coronary artery recanalization with combined bolus injection of recombinant tissue-type plasminogen activator and monoclonal antiplatelet GPIIb/IIIa antibody in a canine preparation. *Circulation* 1988;**77**:670–677.

143. Thompson CM, Steinhubl SR. Monitoring of platelet function in the setting of GPIIb/IIIa inhibitor therapy. *Curr Interv Cardiol Rep* 1999;**1**:270-277.
144. Wheeler GL, Braden GA, Steinhubl SR, Kereiakes DJ, Kottke-Marchant K, Michelson AD, Furman MI, Mueller MN, Moliterno DJ, Sane DC. The Ultegra rapid platelet-function assay: comparison to standard platelet function assays in patients undergoing percutaneous coronary intervention with abciximab therapy. *Am Heart J* 2002;**143**:602–611.
145. Simon DI, Liu CB, Ganz P, Kirshenbaum JM, Piana RN, Rogers C, Selwyn AP, Popma JJ. A comparative study of light transmission aggregometry and automated bedside platelet function assays in patients undergoing percutaneous coronary intervention and receiving abciximab, eptifibatide, or tirofiban. *Catheter Cardiovasc Interv* 2001;**52**:425–432.
146. Steinhubl SR, Talley JD, Braden GA, Tcheng JE, Casterella PJ, Moliterno DJ, Navetta FI, Berger PB, Popma JJ, Dangas G, Gallo R, Sane DC, Saucedo JF, Jia G, Lincoff AM, Theroux P, Holmes DR, Teirstein PS, Kereiakes DJ. Point-of-care measured platelet inhibition correlates with a reduced risk of an adverse cardiac event after percutaneous coronary intervention: results of the GOLD (AU-Assessing Ultegra) multicenter study. *Circulation* 2001;**103**:2572–2578.
147. Hezard N, Metz D, Nazeyrollas P, Droulle C, Elaerts J, Potron G, Nguyen P. Use of the PFA-100 apparatus to assess platelet function in patients undergoing PTCA during and after infusion of c7E3 Fab in the presence of other antiplatelet agents. *Thromb Haemost* 2000;**83**:540–544.
148. Madan M, Berkowitz SD, Christie DJ, Jennings LK, Smit AC, Sigmon KN, Glazer S, Tcheng JE. Rapid assessment of glycoprotein IIb/IIIa blockade with the platelet function analyzer (PFA-100) during percutaneous coronary intervention. *Am Heart J* 2001;**141**:226–233.
149. Madan M, Berkowitz SD, Christie DJ, Smit AC, Sigmon KN, Tcheng JE. Determination of platelet aggregation inhibition during percutaneous coronary intervention with the platelet function analyzer PFA-100. *Am Heart J* 2002;**144**:151–158.

6 Platelet Genomics

Brian K. Jefferson, Kandice Kottke-Marchant and
Eric J. Topol

Introduction

The old view of the platelet as an inert player with little genetic activity after leaving the parent megakaryocyte is no longer accurate. Instead, platelets are regarded now as dynamic components of the thrombotic process, able to continuously synthesize proteins and adapt rapidly to the changing circulatory environment as they are needed in vascular injury. After injury, platelet glycoprotein receptors bind to the exposed subendothelial matrix proteins such as collagen and von Willebrand Factor (vWF).[1,2] After adhesion and tethering to the damaged substrate, platelets become activated and up-regulate glycoprotein surface receptors and release local factors such as adenosine diphosphate (ADP) and cellular vWF.[3] This complex cascade of events results in platelet-platelet interactions between platelet glycoprotein (GP) receptors and fibrinogen and ultimately leads to the thrombus formation. The critical role of platelets in this process requires them to react quickly to form a hemostatic plug to control possible life threatening injuries. Unfortunately, when this process goes awry pathologic thrombosis may occur and lead to development of such diseases as acute myocardial infarction and deep venous thrombosis.

The recent sequencing of the human genome is one of the greatest achievements in the history of western science. Insights gained from the genome project have led to a better understanding of normal physiology and disease states. Understanding of the genetic defects involved in various cardiovascular diseases such as myocardial infarction,[4] long QT syndrome.[5] and hypertrophic cardiomyopathy[6,7] have led to treatments options for people suffering from these diseases. Along with the sequencing of the genome have come powerful tools for molecular analysis. However, application of these tools and the information gained from the genome project to the study of platelet genetics has posed some difficulty. Platelets are anucleate thus lacking their own nuclear DNA. In the past, analysis of platelet genetics has relied largely on the analysis of mutations or functional polymorphism in the platelet surface receptors and correlation of these genetic mutations to clinical disease states and functional changes in platelet biology. Genetic mutations leading to altered function or even complete lack of surface receptors, such as the absence of the glycoprotein IIbIIIa receptor seen with Glanzmann's thrombasthenia or lack of glycoprotein Ib/V/IX receptor with Bernard-Soulier disease, are rare but well-known causes of abnormal platelet function and inherited bleeding disorders.[8] Characterization of these mutations in the receptor genetic sequences have led to a better understanding of platelet function in normal hemostasis as well as bleeding disorders resulting from these mutations.

Better understanding of the genetic mutations leading to abnormal platelet function and the underlying processes of platelet transcription and translation has led to a more complete understanding of the role of the platelet in health and disease. This chapter will cover the progress of platelet genomics from the characterization of multiple platelet receptor polymorphisms to the rapidly evolving fields of platelet genomics and proteomics. Additionally, it will provide the reader a general overview of many of the molecular techniques and methods which will play an increasingly important role in the diagnosis and development of novel treatments for human thrombotic disease in the future.

Platelet Surface Receptor Polymorphisms

Single nucleotide polymorphisms (SNPs) are single base substitutions resulting from mutation of one nucleotide for another in a DNA sequence. Between individuals, the genomes, with respect to base pairs, are 99.9% identical.[9] Thus, only a minute fraction of the human genome is responsible for the variability between individuals in normal health and disease. These differences in the makeup of the genetic code are responsible for the uniqueness of each individual, such as eye color, height and the underlying predisposition for various disease states. These inherent differences account for our varied responses to environmental and pharmacologic stimuli. Of the ten million SNPs in the human genome, only a small fraction is associated with functional significance and the genesis of complex traits. Overlaid on the complexity of the entire human genome, SNPs serve as a compass to help recognize target areas that may contribute to the elementary mechanisms leading to pathologic states.

Genetic association studies are statistical analyses of the relationships between SNP alleles and the phenotypic differences seen in a population of individuals. The overall power of this type of association analysis is a direct function of the number and quality of the SNPs used to screen a population for phenotypic variability and the ability to accurately specify the observed phenotype. For this reason, large databases of SNPs have been developed along with improved methods to screen immense numbers of SNP candidates. As with any observation study methodology, there are some important limitations with SNP studies. Risk association with a particular SNP alone does not provide evidence that the candidate SNP has functional consequences. Additionally, virtually all SNP studies are flawed by incomplete cataloging of the candidate genes. Most SNP studies then represent a limited view of the gene of interest. Furthermore, by using an *a priori* "candidate" approach, SNPs of a potential interest represent a bias of the investigators as to what gene(s) may be implicated. Other deficient issues seen in most SNP association studies include the need to define functional significance underlying the mutation and difficulties often seen replicating the significance in separate populations (Table 1).

Observed associations between a SNP and a particular phenotype may be due to a primary effect on the gene product or may result from linkage with nearby genes. Haplotypes are a block of SNPs that combine to exert a biologic susceptibility to the condition. In complex disease states, haplotype analysis may help overcome some of the limitations of single SNP analysis. Both SNPs and haplotypes can vary significantly in their prevalence among different geographic or ethnic populations. A SNP

Table 1. Platelet components with suggested polymorphism effect on cardiovascular diseases.

Gene/Protein	Ref. No(s).
GPIbα	
GPIIIa	
GPIIb	
GPVI	
Integrin α2	
FCγRIIa	
vWF	60, 143, 144
PECAM	145–147
P-Selectin	148
PDGF	149
α2 adrenergic receptor	150–152
P2Y12 ADP receptor	
P2Y1 ADP receptor	
P2X1 ADP receptor	
TGFβ	153–155

associated with a particular disease in one population will not likely have the same frequency or effect in another population. Further, linkage disequilibrium differs between populations and lack of replication between populations does not necessarily refute the finding of an association. To overcome these limitations and lend credibility to studies, comparison of the prevalence of genetic markers in subjects with a given condition with prevalence in controls needs adequate samples both in number and heterogeneity.

After vascular endothelial injury platelet surface glycoprotein receptors bind to exposed subendothelial extracellular matrix proteins such as vWF and collagen. The adhesion of platelets to the subendothelium subsequently leads to platelet activation with upregulation of other platelet surface glycoprotein receptors, degranulation of the platelet contents such as ADP, clotting factors, and vWF, and subsequent platelet aggregation leading to thrombosis. It is logical that genetic variability in platelet surface receptors might modulate platelet adhesion or aggregative abilities and lead to altered susceptibilities to platelet-mediated thrombosis. Multiple mutations in platelet surface receptors and components with suggested impact on cardiovascular pathologies have been characterized[10–13] (Table 1). Due at least, in part, to the above limitations in SNP analysis, many of the risk association studies for these mutations in CAD and MI have met with controversy with attempts to replicate findings in separate or larger populations. Thus, despite many suggestive findings, these analyses are generally preliminary and hypothesis-generating in nature and should always be interpreted in the context of these limitations.

Specific Receptor Polymorphisms

GP Ia-IIa

The integrin $\alpha_2\beta_1$, or glycoprotein IaIIa, is one of two collagen receptors on the platelet surface. Upon stimulation by collagen binding, the receptor undergoes change from low affinity to high affinity state. Expression of this receptor on the cell surface varies up to threefold among the normal population. This variability has been connected to inheritance of several allelic polymorphisms within the coding sequence of the α_2 gene.[14,15] Allele 1, 807T/1648G/2531C is associated with higher levels of $\alpha_2\beta_1$ while two other alleles (807/C/1648G/2531C) and (807C/1648A/2531C) are each associated with lower levels of the receptor.[16,17] *In vitro* studies have shown that the changes in receptor density may correlate with rates of adhesion to fibrillar collagen under shear conditions.[14]

Multiple studies looking at the C807T mutation have suggested a link between the 807T allele resulting in higher receptor density and complications from arterial thromboic disease.[18–21] In a case control study of 177 patients and 89 matched controls, Moshfegh *et al.* described a three-fold higher prevalence (16.4% versus 5.6%, $p = 0.022$) for those homozygous for the 807T genotype.[18] Santoso *et al.* observed similar adverse impact of the C807T dimorphism in younger patients in a cohort of 2000 male patients undergoing coronary angiography (Age < 49 years; odds ratio, 2.61; $p = 0.009$).[20] Similar reports revealing a negative impact of carriers of the dimorphism and increased risk of CVA and diabetic retinopathy have also been reported although there are conflicting data.[22–24]

GP IIbIIIa

The integrin $\alpha_{IIb}\beta_3$ is the most abundant receptor on the platelet surface (80,000/per platelet) with the surface density increasing upon platelet activation.[13,25] Stable adhesion of the growing thrombus occurs as this receptor binds to both immobilized fibrin/fibrinogen and vWF in the final common pathway in thrombus formation. The most common and best characterized mutation, occurring in approximately 15% of the Caucasian population, is a polymorphism at residue 33 of the β_3 subunit (Leu33Pro).[26] The wild type variant of the β_3 subunit, is often referred to as PLA1 or HPA-1a while the variant (Pro33) is often referred to as PLA2 or HPA-1b.[27] PLA2 is associated with post-transfusion purpura and neonatal alloimmune thrombocytopenia with alloantibodies forming against the A1 allele.[28,29]

In a provocative study of platelet polymorphisms, Weiss *et al.* reported that the gene frequency of the PLA2 allele was over three fold higher in young patients with myocardial infarction or unstable angina when compared to controls.[30] Similar to most polymorphisms in platelet surface receptors, there are multiple subsequent conflicting reports showing both positive and negative associations with ischemic atherosclerotic disease. In an array-based multiplex analysis of 12 candidate polymorphisms, the PLA2 as well as the 4 GF polymorphism of PAI1 was associated with an increased risk of myocardial infarction, suggesting that PLA2 may be risk for thrombosis but not atherosclerosis.[31] Two autopsy studies have shown the Pro33 variant to be associated with coronary thrombus.[32,33] Interestingly, increased plasma fibrinogen levels have been correlated with an increased risk of cardiovascular events in PLA2 carriers (HR = 2.7; 95% CI, 1.1 to 7.1; $p = 0.03$ in the highest quartile of fibrinogen levels).[34] This interaction may account for some of the discrepancies noted in some association studies. No significant association of the PLA2 polymorphism with venous thrombosis or peripheral vascular disease and only a very weak suggestion of association with cerebral vascular disease.[35–42]

There are no clear mechanistic data underlying the effect of the PLA2 mutation on platelet function. *Ex vivo* studies examining effect of the mutation on stimulated platelets are inconsistent in their findings.[43–48] Cell lines expressing Pro33 show enhanced shear stress binding to fibrinogen and abnormal migratory behavior on extracellular matrix substrates.[49,50] These effects may be due to increases in downstream phosphorylation from more efficient outside-in signaling.[51]

Glycoprotein Ib-V-IX

The glycoprotein Ib-V-IX complex plays a central role in mediating platelet adhesion and interaction with the sub-endothelium under conditions of high shear stress.[52,53] It is the second most abundant platelet surface glycoprotein receptor, with approximately 25,000 copies/platelet. The largest subunit of the glycoprotein complex, GP1α (135 kd), contains multiple binding sites for other constituents important in thrombosis and thrombus stabilization such as vWF, α-thrombin and the RGD sequence of the IIβIIIα receptor.[12,54] Thus, GP Ib-V-IX is central to all phases of thrombosis from adhesion through activation and aggregation.

Three main polymorphic sites in the Ibα gene have been attributed to an increased risk for thrombotic events.[54–57] The Thr145Met mutation is responsible for the Ko epitopes (HPA-2) and is in linkage disequilibrium with the variable number tandem repeat (VNTR) polymorphisms in the macroglycopeptide region of GPIbα. The VNTR region results in the duplication of a 13-amino acid sequence of GPIbα. A small number of studies have demonstrated an increased risk between Met145 (VNTR A or B) and risk of prevalence and severity of CAD while others report no association.[58–60] Additionally, no association of the VNTR A or B was seen with MI in young patients or ischemic cerebrovascular events.[35,61–63] *In vitro* studies of the receptor variants have shown no association to platelet aggregation variation in response to ristocetin or botrocetin for both isoforms Met145 and Thr145.[64,65]

The Kozak polymorphism of the GPIbα gene is a T/C dimorphism at nucleotide-5 located in the translation initiation codon of the GPIbα gene.[66,67] The -5C allele is associated with increased translational efficiency of GPIbα mRNA and increased levels of the receptor on the platelet surface.[66] In over 1000 patients with acute coronary syndromes from the OPUS-TIMI 16 trial, the -5C variant was associated with an increased risk of MI.[68] However, the majority of trials have shown no association with any of the Kozak variants.[23,67,69]

GP VI and the Fc receptor

Glycoprotein VI is a 63 kd transmembrane glycoprotein that associates with the platelet Fc receptor and serves as the primary collagen signaling receptor in the platelet.[12,70] Croft *et al.* described five SNPs in the exons of the GP VI gene that result in AA substitutions.[71] In a case-control study on inpatients with MI, one SNP, Ser219Pro, was associated with an increased risk of MI. A second study of 1456 patients with MI in Japan also found an increased risk with another GP VI SNP Thr249Ala.[72] A third SNP had no association with CVA in Australian individuals.[73] The Fc receptor exists as two isoforms His131 and Arg131.[10] Several studies have correlated heparin induced thrombocytopenia to be associated with the Arg131 isoform.[74] This isoform is postulated to reduce clearance of immune complexes causing prolonged activation of platelets leading to pathologic thrombosis.[75]

Platelet ADP receptors

Adenosine diphosphate (ADP) plays a crucial role in hemostasis and thrombosis as a powerful platelet agonist.[76] There are three characterized platelet ADP receptors: 2 G-protein linked receptors — the Gi linked P2Y12 receptor and the Gq linked P2Y1 receptor — and a ligand gated ion channel P2X1 receptor. The P2X1 receptor induces transmembrane Ca^{++} flux in response to ADP but does not appear to play a central role in platelet aggregation[77] P2Y12 is associated with inhibition of adenyl cyclase, platelet activation, thrombus growth and thrombus stability, and P2Y1 is associated with the activation of PLC, platelet shape change and intracellular calcium mobilization. Inhibition of either receptor prevents platelet aggregation.[76,78]

Fontana *et al.* catalogued haplotypes in the P2Y12 receptor associated with abnormal platelet aggregation in response to ADP induced platelet aggregation.[79] In their study, one particular haplotype, H2, was significantly associated with a higher degree of ADP induced platelet aggregation. Further, in a case-control study of 172 males with peripheral arterial disease, the H2 haplotype was more frequent in subjects with PAD ($OR = 2.3$, $p = 0.002$) after multivariate analysis. This haplotype showed no association with abnormal tissue factor expression or platelet response to the

P2Y12 antagonist clopidogrel. Further cataloging of the P2Y12 gene has shown more extensive dimorphic variation than previously described. None of these variations were associated with abnormal response to ADP in a cohort of patients taking aspirin (unpublished data).

Multiple polymorphisms exist in the P2Y1 gene. Hetherington *et al.* described a silent dimorphism in the P2Y1 gene, 1622AG associated with abnormal response to ADP induced platelet activation.[80] Our group reported another SNP in the P2Y1 gene to be associated with abnormal platelet function in response to arachidonic acid induced platelet aggregation.[81] While little is known about the P2X1 variations, Greco *et al.* reported expression of a deletion mutation of the P2X1 receptor that may preferentially be activated by ADP.[82]

Platelet Surface Receptor Polymorphisms and Pharmacogenomics

Arterial thrombotic complications of atherosclerotic disease are the leading cause of mortality in western society. Platelets play a pivotal role in this process and antiplatelet therapies have had a huge impact on preventing complications and improving survival from myocardial infarction and stroke. Unfortunately, these therapies often carry significant side effects, and therapies that may be life saving in one individual may have no benefit or be frankly harmful in another. These risks are magnified as we are progressing to an era where many of these medications are administered concurrently. With the increasing number of antithrombotic agents available, the concomitant use of one or more of these medications will require maximizing benefits of each, while reducing the overall risks of multiple therapies. An understanding of who benefits from these medications prior to their administration will play an important role in reducing the risk. The three most significant antiplatelet therapies currently used in cardiovascular medicine today are aspirin, clopidogrel, and glycoprotein IIb/IIIa inhibitors. Clinical response to of each these therapies have been associated with platelet genetic variation. As in other SNP association studies, consistent independent replication has been a central issue when applying the associative risk to larger clinical populations.

Aspirin

Although aspirin is a relatively weak antiplatelet drug based on platelet aggregation testing, it is one of the first-line therapeutic options in the treatment of cardiovascular disease.[83] Several clinical trials have proven its efficacy in primary and secondary prevention of occlusive cardiovascular events.[84,85] Aspirin exerts its effect by blocking only one of the pathways that lead to platelet aggregation, by irreversibly inactivating cyclooxygenase-1 (COX-1) which is necessary for the conversion of arachidonic acid to thromboxane A2. This ultimately stimulates platelet aggregation and vascular constriction. COX-2 is inducible by other pathways, and is incompletely inhibited by aspirin's effects and provides an alternative pathway for thromboxane synthesis. Studies have shown that approximately 8%–45% of individuals are aspirin resistant[86,87] and resistance is associated with poor clinical outcomes.[88] The incidence has recently been questioned and attributed to compliance issues and methodology of assessment.[89] However, several studies have correlated genetic predisposition with lack of aspirin pharmacologic effect.

The PLA2 dimorphism has been associated with a reduced response to aspirin therapy. *Ex vivo* studies of platelet function have shown that the PLA2 is associated with abnormal response to platelet agonist including reduced thrombin generation and inhibition of collagen induced aggregation.[90,91] Several groups have tied clinical thrombotic predisposition while on aspirin therapy to carriers of the PLA2 polymorphism. Walter *et al.* reported an over five fold increase in intracoronary stent thrombosis to carriers of the mutant allele.[92] Other reports have supported this observation, but to a lesser degree.[93,94]

We demonstrated a single base substitution in the P2Y1 platelet ADP receptor to be associated with more than a three fold increase in clinical aspirin resistance.[81] Heatherington *et al.* demonstrated a genetic component to abnormal response to ADP.[80] With the large number of patients using aspirin for both primary and secondary prevention of cardiovascular events, further studies are needed to elaborate additional genetic predispositions that may cause decreased benefit of this important therapy.

Glycoprotein IIb/IIIa inhibitors

GP IIbIIIa antagonists are qualitatively different from classical antiplatelet agents, such as aspirin or clopidogrel as they do not primarily inhibit platelet signal generation but instead act outside the platelet through competition for ligand (e.g. fibrinogen, vWF) receptors that are essential for platelet bridging and aggregate formation. These agents have shown significant benefit when used as adjuvant therapies in the treatment of acute coronary syndromes.[95] Three intravenous compounds are currently in clinical use: abciximab, an antibody fragment, and two low-molecular weight compounds, tirofiban and eptifibatide.

Several studies have suggested an interaction with the PLA2 polymorphism and abnormal *ex vivo* and clinical platelet responses to these agents.[96,97] However, there are significant conflicting data. PLA2 was associated with reduced bleeding complications in a large scale prospective clinical trial of chronic preventive therapy with oral IIbIIIa inhibition.[98] Future studies of antiplatelet therapies may need to take into account genomic identification of those receiving benefit or excess risk from these medications especially as alternate adjuvant therapies such as direct thrombin inhibitors and intravenous P2Y12 antagonist become available.

P2Y12 inhibitors

Dual antiplatelet therapy with aspirin and P2Y12 inhibition, primarily with clopidogrel, is now a mainstay for prevention of complications of atherosclerotic disease[99,100] It is generally accepted in clinical practice that the response to clopidogrel therapy is variable among the population and that some patients do not receive adequate inhibition from standard use of this medication.[101] However, clopidogrel resistance is a poorly defined entity with no clear assay to assess platelet response to clopidogrel therapy, especially for those on dual antiplatelet therapies. Gurbel *et al.* reported that 25% of patients displayed a lack of clopidogrel effect on platelet aggregation after coronary stenting.[102] Polymorphisms in the P2Y12 receptor have also been linked to lack of ADP induced platelet aggregation.[103] With dual antiplatelet therapy now showing benefit on a long term basis, defining the populations that receive maximal benefit from these agents will become increasingly important.

Genomic Analysis in Platelets

In SNP association studies, specific gene candidates are identified and evaluated for association with a particular phenotype. In a genome wide scan, approximately 400 short tandem repeat markers (microsatellites) evenly spaced every 10 cM across the genome are assessed to hunt for a linkage peak of common alleles across subjects with a prespecified phenotype. The peaks of DNA identified by the microsatellite markers may fluctuate among a phenotype and thus serve as a signal of genetic variation. This variability can be used to specify regions of interest in the genome that may be in proximity to the gene or genes responsible for a particular phenotype. Further fine mapping of the region of interest must then take place to identify the locus responsible for the phenotype. Using this approach, Drachman *et al.* identified a specific locus on the short arm of chromosome 10 with a maximum two-point lod score of 5.68 in a family with autosomal dominant thrombocytopenia.[104] In another scan using microsatellite markers covering the X chromosome, Mehaffey *et al.* identified a novel mutation the *GATA-1* gene, which encodes a transcription factor involved in megakaryocyte development responsible for a pedigree of X-linked thrombocytopenia.[105] Quantitative trait mapping has shown linkage peaks for platelet count at several loci in human and murine analyses.[106,107]

Novel Methods for Platelet Genomic Analysis

The availability of large scale genomic databases and libraries have led to a better understanding of the underlying molecular pathogenesis of complex diseases such as myocardial infarction, increased facilitation of risk of disease and identified many new and useful therapeutic targets. As platelets are lacking nuclear DNA, traditional methods of genetic analysis such as genome wide scanning are somewhat limited in examining platelet genetics. While the elucidation of many platelet receptor SNPs has led to a better understanding of platelet function and pathogenesis, these approaches lack true applicability as they do not address the multitude of changes that platelets experience as they transition from a quiescent state through activation and thrombosis. Also, with much of the underlying relevant platelet physiology and pathology occurring through the myriad of events after the initiation of cellular activation, other approaches of genetic analysis may be more fruitful in identifying potential targets.

Traditional genomic approaches lack the ability to detect changes of transcriptional and translational activity, alternative protein isoforms, critical protein interactions, and are unable to identify important post-translational modifications that ultimately lead to thrombosis. However, the availability of powerful genetic databases for genomic analysis and the development of more efficient molecular analysis tools and software have facilitated better characterization of the platelet genetics through further characterization of the platelet proteome and transcriptome.

Platelet Proteomics

The proteome of an organism is defined as the total protein complement of the genome at a given time and is comprised of thousands of diverse proteins that change in time and expression depending on the underlying state of the cell.[108] At any given time, more than 10,000 genes can be expressed in a single cell. Each of these genes can further undergo extensive regulation at the transcriptional, translational and post-translational levels resulting in potentially millions of different protein components expressed. Thus, the proteome of the organism is ever changing with an infinite number of possible variations. Proteomics is the application of global approaches to identify and assess protein function and expression in the cell.

Current approaches to evaluate cellular protein dynamics incorporate multiple techniques of protein analysis, some of which have been used for decades. Protein improvements in separation by two-dimensional electrophoresis or multidimensional chromatography, differential image analysis and mass spectrometric analysis, coupled to expressed tag sequence databases have resulted in the ability to characterize thousands of proteins have advanced the field of proteomics. Several comprehensive proteomic maps are now available, such as the interactive web site SWISS-PROT 2-D

PAGE and the 2-10 2-DE map by Marcus *et al.*[109,110] However, the field of platelet proteomics is still relatively young and although large proteomic maps are published, the overall number of proteins characterized is still relatively small.

Methods of proteomic analysis

High resolution two-dimensional electrophoresis (2-DE) separates proteins in two dimensions based on two independent properties of the proteins and is one of the most often used techniques for protein analysis. This method separates proteins according to their isoelectric point in one dimension and then separates them into a second dimension based on their molecular mass.[111–113] The result is a characteristic map with a distinctive protein spot profile for each cell type. These protein profiles can then be compared to known protein spot patterns identified by using the same separation conditions with specialized imaging software and known proteomic databases. Novel or unidentified spots can then be excised from the others and digested with sequence specific proteases to allow further identification.

Previous limitations with the gels used for separation have been overcomed through the development of narrow pH range gels and isoelectric focusing, greatly increasing the resolution and reproducibility of 2-DE. A second method of protein separation uses multiple liquid orthogonal chromatography coupled to mass spectrometry where proteins are separated by charge using a cation exchange resin followed by charge separation with reverse phase high pressure liquid chromatography. This method is more amenable to automation and detects proteins not easily separated using 2-DE.[111,114,115]

Mass spectrometry (MS) is central to the field of proteomics and is the only way that protein candidates can be rapidly identified with any degree of specificity and sensitivity.[116] MS is an indirect method of protein analysis which measures the mass to charge ratio after a charge is applied by a variety of methods to the protein. Basic mass spectrometers consist of three parts. The first is an ionization source which converts molecules into gas phase ions. Once created, the ions are separated by a second device called the mass analyzer. The mass analyzer separates ions of variable mass charge ratios based on electric or magnetic fields, or time of flight (TOF) which are then transferred to an ion detector. The largest improvements in MS have come with the development of techniques to create ions of large molecules such as proteins. MALDI (Matrix Assisted Laser Desorption Ionization) creates ions by excitation of the molecules isolated from the energy of the laser through an energy absorbing matrix. The proteins separated using either 2-DE or liquid chromatography are excised and enzymatically digested into peptide fragments or eluted from the cation exchange resin directly onto a mass spectrometer. The resulting profile from mass spectrometer can then be compared to multiple available protein and peptide databases for exact identification. Further analysis can lead to direct protein sequencer identification using techniques that generate amino acid sequence data for each protein.

Platelet proteomics can be used to generate expression maps for the entire complement of proteins expressed at any given time in a platelet, to analyze the changes in platelet protein expression due to external influences, or platelet protein-protein interactions. Variations in protein expression or unidentified proteins can be compared to available genomic databases to identify genes and mutations responsible for particular phenotypes.

Identification of platelet proteins using proteomics

While recent improvements in methodologies have advanced our knowledge of the platelet proteome, 2-DE has been used to analyze the platelet proteins for over 30 years. Initial experiments using SDS-PAGE led to identification of many of the platelet glycoprotein receptors.[108] Gravel *et al.* used 2-DE map and immunoblotting to identify over 25 proteins from cytosolic and enriched-membrane platelet proteins.[117] Unfortunately, before the use of MS to identify proteins and peptide fragments, time consuming and cumbersome techniques such as N-terminal sequencing were required to sequence proteomic targets. This limited the breadth of the proteomic maps and number of proteins able to be analyzed.

Marcus *et al.* described a cytosolic platelet proteome map (pI 3-10) and identified 186 proteins, mostly cytoskeletal proteins, separated with 2-DE and identified with MALDI-TOF MS.[110] In one of the more comprehensive analyses of the platelet proteome to date, O'Neil *et al.* used broad and narrow range pI to generate a high resolution protein map of 2300 different protein spots. Of the 536 proteins in the 4–5 pI range, 284 acidic proteins were identified using high throughput q-TOF mass spectrometry.[118] These 284 proteins corresponded to 123 different reading frames including six novel proteins. The identified proteins encompassed a wide variety of functionalities with almost 50% encompassing cytoskeletal and signaling proteins (Fig. 1). Also, included in the mix were a large number of transcription factors and centromeric proteins with unknown significance. In a follow-up study, Garcia *et al.* extended a similar analysis to the pI 4–11 region.[119] Seven hundred and sixty proteins from this region were identified, corresponding to 311 different genes and resulting in annotation of 54% of the pI 4–11 range 2-DE proteome map. The main groups of proteins in this range appear to be involved in intracellular signaling and regulation of the cytoskeleton (Fig. 2).

Other useful analyses of proteomic data have come from comparing the proteome using differential analysis between activated and control platelets. Thrombin is one of the most powerful activators of platelets and *in vitro* TRAP is able to activate platelets in a thrombin analogous manner.

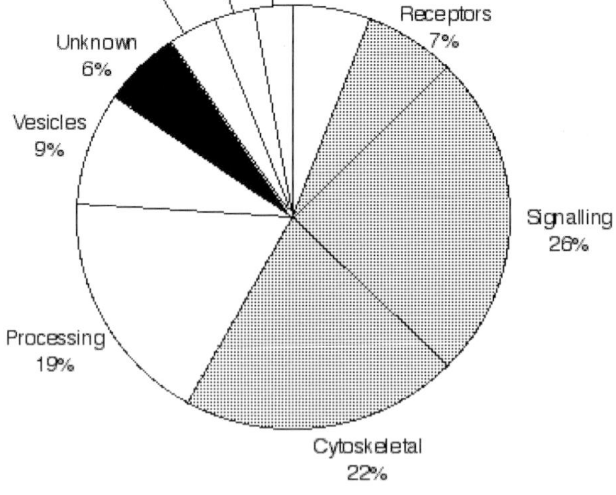

Fig. 1. Categories of protein function isolated in the acidic proteome. Adapted with permission from O'Neill *et al.*[118]

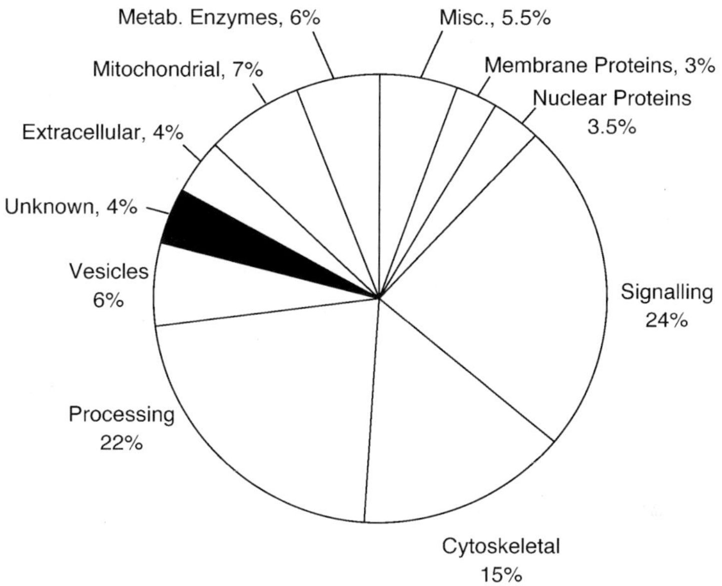

Fig. 2. Categories of protein function isolated from the platelet proteome in the 4–11 pI range. Adapted with permission from Garcia *et al.*[119]

Garcia *et al.* evaluated signaling responses in platelets activated by thrombin receptor activating protein (TRAP) using 2-DE and liquid-chromatography coupled tandem mass spectrometry.[120] These experiments identified over 60 differentially regulated protein features, from which 41 were identified with LCMS/MS including eight previously unreported in platelets. Other important insights from this study includes: (1) identification of several important phosphorylation targets including the adaptor downstream of tyrosine kinase-2 (Dok-2) and RGS 18 and (2) correlation of these downstream phosphorylation events with outside-in-signaling through IIbIIIa and GPVI. Similar approaches have been used to analyze the secretome from thrombin activated platelets.[121] (Fig. 3).

The incorporation of proteomics to identify novel platelet proteins provides a powerful tool. Future directions to identify potential changes in platelet protein expression in patients with pathologic thrombosis or to monitor protein products to assess the efficacy of drug therapy will increase as these methodologies and techniques evolve. Combining the techniques of high throughput genetic analysis with protein analysis have already

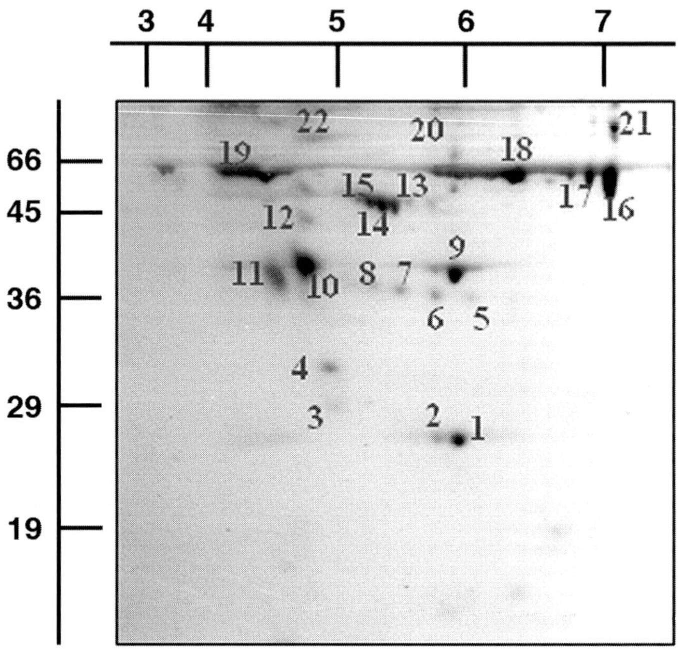

Fig. 3. Representative gel for the two-dimensional electrophoresis of the releasate fraction from thrombin activated platelets. Reproduced with permission from Coppinger *et al.*[121]

yielded significant results as will be further discussed later in this chapter. Current limitations of the proteomic approach include difficulty in protein quantification and detection of smaller peptides, poor correlation of protein expression with levels of cDNA, difficulty observing minor protein constituents and difficulties in examining membrane bound proteins. Methodologies such as mass code affinity tagging coupled to MS, differential florescence tagging, and combination with genetic databases will help overcome many of these limitations and allow more efficient evaluation of protein expression.

Platelet Transcription

Thrombopoesis in the bone marrow results in the generation of platelets from cytoplasmic buds which are released from megakaryocytes and assume a lifespan of approximately ten days in the circulation.[122] Since platelets are formed from the megakaryocytic cytoplasm, they are anucleate and do not contain nuclear DNA. The lack of nuclear material means that the platelet itself is unable to replicate, transcribe nuclear DNA or further regulate message at the transcriptional level. Platelets contain mitochondrial DNA which encodes 13 mRNAs and two rRNAs.[123,124] Newly formed platelets contain larger quantities of mRNA than mature platelets. In the quiescent state, platelets generally display minimal translational activity but contain RNA message for many platelet proteins such as the Fc receptors and protein kinase C isoforms.[125] RNA in platelets was long regarded as a remnant of protein synthesis from the megakaryocyte and not thought to play a significant role in platelet function once they leave the bone marrow. However, stimulation of platelets by agonists such as ADP or through various interactions between platelet surface receptors such as GP IIb/IIIa, GP Ib-V-IX and other integrins within the extracellular matrix after endothelial injury increases platelet protein translation.[125,126] Thus, platelets have multiple levels of potential translational regulation: during thrombopoeisis in the bone marrow and after platelet activation from various platelet agonists. While platelets have long been thought to be a bystander cell, with little synthetic activity forming a "dumb" brick in the ultimate thrombus, the converse is true. They are dynamic participants of the thrombotic process, with active changes occurring at the translational level.

Platelet mRNA is synthesized in the megakaryocyte in a regulated efficient manner and the platelet itself contains thousands of megakaryocyte derived messages. Platelet mRNA is functional and contains the same primary structural aspects as all eukaryotic mRNA including a 5′ cap and 3′poly-A tail.[127,128] Platelets also carry rRNA and the large ribonucleoprotein complexes from which ribosomes are formed and protein synthesis occurs. Ribosomes removed from platelets in a cell free system are able to regulate protein synthesis.[129] Most eukaryotic cell ribosomes are primarily associated with the rough endoplasmic reticulum. In contrast, ribosomes in platelets are primarily associated with the contractile proteins comprising the cytoskeletal framework of the platelet.[129,130] This targets protein synthesis in a strategic geographic location in the platelet. Newly synthesized platelets contain a larger amount of rough endoplasmic reticulum and display a larger capacity for protein synthesis then maturing platelets.[131]

Platelets contain spliceosomes, snRNA and splicing proteins and post-initiation regulation of platelet protein synthesis can occur.[122,126] In response to surface receptor activation, platelets have been shown to excise introns from interleukin 1-β pre-mRNA.[132] Platelet protein translation is also controlled by a variety of numerous other proteins and other small regulatory RNAs. Regulation of protein synthesis at the translational level does carry some advantages especially in a cell that is required to act fast in response to vascular injury and in the control of hemorrhage. Bypassing the steps required in RNA synthetic delay in transcription and primarily controlling protein synthesis at the translation level facilitates this necessarily rapid response.

Historically, the low levels of mRNA in the platelet made studies of gene expression difficult. Platelet RNA analysis was performed with northern blot hybridization and rt-PCR with cDNA library construction. With the further advent of PCR technologies and subsequent improvements in the efficiency of molecular methodologies it is now possible to evaluate both low levels of RNA message and the dynamic changes involved during platelet activation. The two main methods involved in profiling the mRNA repertoire of the platelet, or platelet transcriptome, are DNA microarray technology and serial analysis of gene expression (SAGE).[125,133,134]

Microarray analysis

A microarray is a small substrate on which a large number of cDNA or oligonucleotides representing portions of genes are bound as discrete spots in a known location on the array. These arrays take advantage of the natural property of DNA to hybridize — for adenine to bind to thymine and cytosine to bind to guanine. A large number of arrays are available commercially or can be generated as a tissue or cell specific library. The substrate tethered nucleic acids on the array are used as a probe for the complementary strand in a mixture of radiolabeled nucleic acids from a biologic sample. The complementary base pair interactions can then measured by the detectible radiolabel. Evaluation of the positive signal on the array can provide a picture of the transcript expression in the cell at a single time point. Comparison of signals from a control and treated sample can be performed to evaluate changes in expression occurring after treatment.

With current technology of substrate generation and the ability to hybridize over a million oligonucleotides to a substrate no larger than a thumbnail, arrays that essentially cover the human genome are now available. Coupled with more efficient biometric software analytical algorithms, routine analysis of expression data for tens of thousands of genes can be performed on a routine basis. Many of the initial problems with microarray analysis, such as those leading to excessive variability and lack of reproducibility have also been overcome with these technological improvements. Detailed expression profiling has been used extensively in the field of oncology enabling successful molecular typing and characterization of various neoplasms.[135–137]

SAGE analysis

The platelet phenotype reflects changes in expression patterns that occur through platelet activation and the complex cascade of events resulting from platelet activation. Single defects in platelet receptors or structures are reflected through the changes in subsequent gene expression. SAGE is a high throughput, high efficiency technique that provides analysis of gene expression patterns and quantitative and comprehensive profiles in a given cell population allowing for the characterization of gene expression patterns in a cell. In contrast to microarray analysis, SAGE does not require *a priori* knowledge of transcript information or availability on the microarray being probed, making it an ideal tool to follow the complex chain of events resulting in platelet thrombosis.

SAGE is based on two principles.[138,139] First, a short oligonucleotide sequence tag of 10 or 11 base pairs contains sufficient information to uniquely identify a transcript. These tags can be used to identify genes and the abundance of their mRNA transcripts. Second, concatenation of short sequence tags enabling the efficient serial analysis of transcripts allows high throughput sequencing. SAGE uses short oligonucleotide tags which are generated from unique positions of each species of mRNA. To synthesize these tags, poly(A) RNA is transcribed into biotyinylated ds-cDNA. Digestion with an anchoring enzyme results in shorter cDNA fragments. The strands are isolated with paramagnetic streptavidin beads and the fragments are divided in half and ligated to two different linkers. Each linker contains a restriction site for a tagging enzyme, the anchoring enzyme overhang, and a PCR priming site. The bound linker-cDNA sequences are digested with the tagging enzyme generating fragments of linker and adhering short cDNA sequence tags. These linker-tags are blunt ended. The two sets of linker tags are ligated to linker-ditag-linker constructs and amplified with PCR by using linker specific primers. The constructs are then digested with the anchoring enzyme, releasing the ditags which are isolated and ligated to concatemers, cloned and sequenced. Automated sequencing of the concatamer SAGE tags allows the identification and quantification of cellular transcripts.

This sequence data is analyzed allowing identification of each gene expressed in the cell and the level of that gene's expression which is a direct function of the frequency that each SAGE tag is found in the cloned multimers. Data from SAGE analysis has been used to identify tumor markers in a variety of neoplasms. Using a large number of tags, genes expressed at low levels can readily be identified making SAGE a convenient technique in platelet mRNA analysis.

Platelet Transcriptome

Profiling the platelet transcriptome carries challenges compared to transcript profiling in other tissues. Platelet preparations are often contaminated with leukocytes and purification is often technically challenging. Platelet preparation of RNA is technically difficult and does not yield large quantities of RNA. Additionally, although it is not uncommon in other microarray studies to have contamination from exogenous tissues/cells, the low levels of cytoplasmic mRNA compared to the amount of RNA in nucleated cells such as leukocytes ($>$10,000 fold) make sample purification imperative to eliminate outside signal contamination.[133] Despite these technical issues, a number of groups have successfully used microarray analysis to identify components of the platelet transcriptome.

Using rigorous methods of leukodepletion and DNA amplification, Rox *et al.* demonstrated that micrograms of platelet-specific cDNA could be isolated from single donors and that their gene expression profiles remained constant over time.[140] Bugert *et al.* used multiple filtration procedures to eliminate leukocyte contamination and PCR amplification of genomic DNA to confirm the absence of nucleated cells in their preparation.[141] From this preparation, microarray hybridization was used to analyze 9850 genes in RNA taken from pooled platelets. This analysis of the platelet transcriptome found 1526 gene transcripts. As expected, there was a high representation of genes encoding receptors and glycoproteins and integrins. The full list of their mRNA platelet profile is available on the internet at www.ma.uni-heidelberg.de/inst/iti/plt_array.xls.

Gnatenko *et al.* used CD45 and leukocyte depletion schemes to achieve a greater than 400-fold decrease in leukocytes in a platelet preparation before analysis on an Affymetrix GeneChip.[124] This analysis of over 12,000 probes maximally identified 2147 platelet expressed transcripts. Using the Affymetrix assigned annotations for each gene, over 20% were involved in metabolism and receptor/signaling (Fig. 4). A high representation of the transcripts encoded actin-related machinery consistent with the fact that 20%–30% of the platelet proteome is composed of actin and actin-related

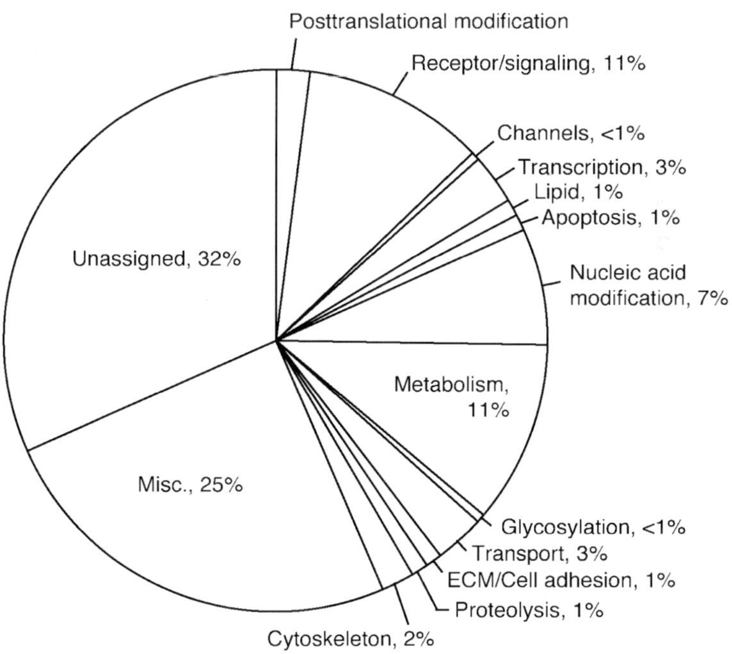

Fig. 4. Relative distribution of platelet expressed genes using microarray analysis. Adapted with permission from Bahou and Gnatenko.[125]

proteins. Validating the power of this type of analysis to identify unique platelet transcripts, was the lack of previous characterization for 50% of the identified transcripts. In order to identify other genes not represented on the microarray, SAGE analysis was performed in parallel. The SAGE demonstrated 2033 tags, of which 89% corresponded to message derived from the mitochondrial DNA. This is not overly surprising given the persistent mitochondrial generation of polyadenylated message through the platelet lifetime enhancing its detection through SAGE. In addition to the mitochondrial transcripts, concordance with the non-mitochondrially derived transcripts identified on both the microarray and SAGE was noted (Fig. 5). Of further interest, from the non-mitochondrial derived tags ($n = 233$) almost 50% were not present on the Affymetrix chip illustrating the complementary power of the two methods in identifying candidates from the platelet transcriptome.

McRedmond *et al.* used the same Affymetrix GeneChip as in the previous study to analyze the transcriptome from a platelet preparation purified with centrifugation.[142] They identified 2928 distinct transcripts from this preparation. Confirming the validity of methods and reproducibility of the microarray technique, 90% of the top 50 genes were shared between the experiments. Similar to the other data, equal proportions of transcripts were seen in each gene annotation cluster in both microarrays. In order to correlate the platelet transcriptome with the platelet proteome, the transcript

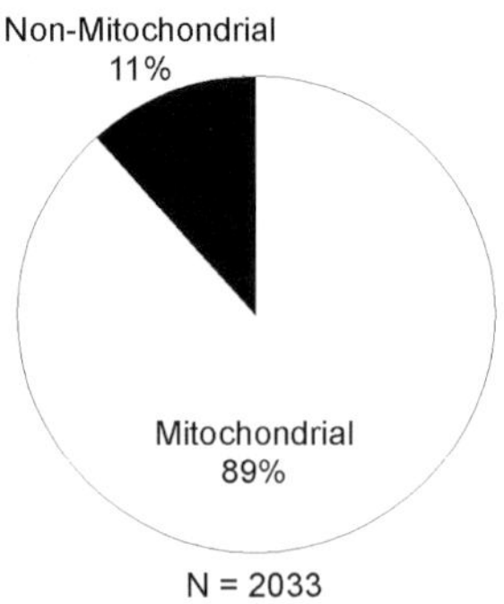

Top 10 Non-Mitochondrial Transcripts

Transcript	No. Tags	Microarray (Rank)
β2-microglobulin	26	+ (9)
Thymosin β4	21	+ (1)
Platelet factor 4	8	+ (8)
Platelet factor 4 variant 1	8	—
β-thromboglobulin	7	+ (22)
Glycoprotein Ibβ	5	+ (13)
H2A histone	3	+ (50)
Cofilin 2	3	+ (47)
Neurogranin	3	+ (2)
Ferritin	3	+ (5)

Fig. 5. Comparative analysis of non-mitochondrial SAGE tags demonstrating strong overall concordance with microarray analysis (+ present, – absent; average rank in parentheses). Adapted with permission from Bahou and Gnatenko.[125]

profiles were compared to an analysis of platelet secreted proteins and the proteomic data from the previously described Marcus and O'Neill proteomic mapping studies.[110,118] From this comparison, 69% of the secreted platelet proteins were detectable at the RNA transcript level with similar results from the other proteomic datasets. Of the 50 most abundant platelet messages, 40% were represented in the platelet releasate. Thus, the platelet transcriptome and the proteome compliment each other and analysis of each may provide novel insight into platelet physiology. Extrapolation of these methods to discover novel mechanisms underlying abnormal platelet pathology may provide important knowledge into new methods of treatment.

Conclusion

Arterial thrombotic disease is the leading cause of morbidity and mortality in western society. Despite knowledge of many modifiable risk factors, the prevalence continues to increase. Clearly, there is an urgent need to correctly identify those patients who are at risk for the often devastating outcomes resulting from pathologic thrombosis. Evaluation and characterization of genetic risk factors such as platelet polymorphisms and haplotypes have led to many promising, yet conflicting results. Analysis of both the platelet proteome and transcriptome are still in the rudimentary phases. It is unclear at this juncture which of these techniques will prove most valuable in elucidating the risk and genetic mechanisms leading to pathologic states, and currently we are without a rapid and clinically fully validated platelet functional assay. This remains a huge obstacle in identifying relevant genes and proteins involved in abnormal platelet physiology. However, with the rapid advances in molecular technologies, large databases cataloging the platelet genome, transcriptome and proteome will facilitate and further our knowledge of platelet function and dysfunction providing a broader knowledge with greater clinical applicability. This new era of medicine poses new challenges for patient confidentiality and ethical decisions for screening those at risk. These challenges will be important to remember in order to successfully identify and treat patients at risk for thrombotic disorders.

References

1. Goto S. Role of von Willebrand factor for the onset of arterial thrombosis. *Clin Lab* 2001;**47**:327–334.
2. Goto S, Salomon DR, Ikeda Y, *et al.* Characterization of the unique mechanism mediating the shear-dependent binding of soluble von Willebrand factor to platelets. *J Biol Chem* 1995;**270**:23352–23361.
3. Packham MA. Role of platelets in thrombosis and hemostasis. *Can J Physiol Pharmacol* 1994;**72**:278–284.
4. Wang L, Fan C, Topol SE, *et al.* Mutation of MEF2A in an inherited disorder with features of coronary artery disease. *Science* 2003;**302**:1578–1581.
5. Antzelevitch C. Molecular genetics of arrhythmias and cardiovascular conditions associated with arrhythmias. *J Cardiovasc Electrophysiol* 2003;**14**:1259–1272.
6. Hughes SE, McKenna WJ. New insights into the pathology of inherited cardiomyopathy. *Heart* 2005;**91**:257–264.
7. Bashyam MD, Savithri GR, Kumar MS, *et al.* Molecular genetics of familial hypertrophic cardiomyopathy (FHC). *J Hum Genet* 2003;**48**:55–64.
8. Nurden AT. Qualitative disorders of platelets and megakaryocytes. *J Thromb Haemost* 2005;**3**:1773–1782.
9. Peters RJ, Boekholdt SM. Gene polymorphisms and the risk of myocardial infarction — an emerging relation. *N Engl J Med* 2002;**347**:1963–1965.
10. Santoso S. Platelet polymorphisms in thrombotic disorders. *Transfus Clin Biol* 2001;**8**:261–266.
11. Kottke-Marchant K. Genetic polymorphisms associated with venous and arterial thrombosis: an overview. *Arch Pathol Lab Med* 2002;**126**:295–304.
12. Yee DL, Bray PF. Clinical and functional consequences of platelet membrane glycoprotein polymorphisms. *Semin Thromb Hemost* 2004;**30**:591–600.
13. Bray PF. Platelet glycoprotein polymorphisms as risk factors for thrombosis. *Curr Opin Hematol* 2000;**7**:284–289.
14. Kritzik M, Savage B, Nugent DJ, *et al.* Nucleotide polymorphisms in the alpha2 gene define multiple alleles that are associated with differences in platelet alpha2 beta1 density. *Blood* 1998;**92**:2382–2388.
15. Kunicki TJ, Kritzik M, Annis DS, *et al.* Hereditary variation in platelet integrin alpha2 beta1 density is associated with two silent polymorphisms in the alpha2 gene coding sequence. *Blood* 1997;**89**:1939–1943.
16. Kalb R, Santoso S, Unkelbach K, *et al.* Localization of the Br polymorphism on a 144 bp exon of the GPIa gene and its application in platelet DNA typing. *Thromb Haemost* 1994;**71**:651–654.

17. Santoso S, Kalb R, Walka M, *et al.* The human platelet alloantigens Br(a) and Brb are associated with a single amino acid polymorphism on glycoprotein Ia (integrin subunit alpha 2). *J Clin Invest* 1993;**92**:2427–2432.
18. Moshfegh K, Wuillemin WA, Redondo M, *et al.* Association of two silent polymorphisms of platelet glycoprotein Ia/IIa receptor with risk of myocardial infarction: a case-control study. *Lancet* 1999;**353**:351–354.
19. Kroll H, Gardemann A, Fechter A, *et al.* The impact of the glycoprotein Ia collagen receptor subunit A1648G gene polymorphism on coronary artery disease and acute myocardial infarction. *Thromb Haemost* 2000;**83**:392–396.
20. Santoso S, Kunicki TJ, Kroll H, *et al.* Association of the platelet glycoprotein Ia C807T gene polymorphism with nonfatal myocardial infarction in younger patients. *Blood* 1999;**93**:2449–2453.
21. Leone AM, De S, V, Burzotta F, *et al.* Glycoprotein Ia C807T gene polymorphism and increased risk of recurrent acute coronary syndromes: a fivc ycar follow up. *Heart* 2004;**90**:567–569.
22. Carlsson LE, Santoso S, Spitzer C, *et al.* The alpha2 gene coding sequence T807/A873 of the platelet collagen receptor integrin alpha2 beta1 might be a genetic risk factor for the development of stroke in younger patients. *Blood* 1999;**93**:3583–3586.
23. Frank MB, Reiner AP, Schwartz SM, *et al.* The Kozak sequence polymorphism of platelet glycoprotein Ibalpha and risk of nonfatal myocardial infarction and nonfatal stroke in young women. *Blood* 2001;**97**:875–879.
24. Reiner AP, Kumar PN, Schwartz SM, *et al.* Genetic variants of platelet glycoprotein receptors and risk of stroke in young women. *Stroke* 2000;**31**:1628–1633.
25. Niiya K, Hodson E, Bader R, *et al.* Increased surface expression of the membrane glycoprotein IIb/IIIa complex induced by platelet activation. Relationship to the binding of fibrinogen and platelet aggregation. *Blood* 1987;**70**:475–483.
26. Santoso S, Kiefel V. Human platelet-specific alloantigens: update. *Vox Sang* 1998;**74**(Suppl 2):249–253.
27. Newman PJ. Nomenclature of human platelet alloantigens: a problem with the HPA system? *Blood* 1994;**83**:1447–1451.
28. Moser R, Fae I, Neumeister A, *et al.* Neonatal allo-immune thrombocytopenia due to fetomaternal HPA-1 incompatibility of a homozygous HPA-1a mother and a homozygous HPA-1b father. A case report. *Eur J Pediatr* 1994;**153**:95–97.
29. Evenson DA, Stroncek DF, Pulkrabek S, *et al.* Posttransfusion purpura following bone marrow transplantation. *Transfusion* 1995;**35**:688–693.

30. Weiss EJ, Bray PF, Tayback M, *et al.* A polymorphism of a platelet glycoprotein receptor as an inherited risk factor for coronary thrombosis. *N Engl J Med* 1996;**334**:1090–1094.
31. Pastinen T, Perola M, Niini P, *et al.* Array-based multiplex analysis of candidate genes reveals two independent and additive genetic risk factors for myocardial infarction in the Finnish population. *Hum Mol Genet* 1998;**7**:1453–1462.
32. Mikkelsson J, Perola M, Laippala P, *et al.* Glycoprotein IIIa Pl(A) polymorphism associates with progression of coronary artery disease and with myocardial infarction in an autopsy series of middle-aged men who died suddenly. *Arterioscler Thromb Vasc Biol* 1999;**19**:2573–2578.
33. Mikkelsson J, Perola M, Penttila A, *et al.* The GPIIIa (beta3 integrin) PlA polymorphism in the early development of coronary atherosclerosis. *Atherosclerosis* 2001;**154**:721–727.
34. Boekholdt SM, Peters RJ, de Maat MP, *et al.* Interaction between a genetic variant of the platelet fibrinogen receptor and fibrinogen levels in determining the risk of cardiovascular events. *Am Heart J* 2004;**147**:181–186.
35. Carlsson LE, Greinacher A, Spitzer C, *et al.* Polymorphisms of the human platelet antigens HPA-1, HPA-2, HPA-3, and HPA-5 on the platelet receptors for fibrinogen (GPIIb/IIIa), von Willebrand factor (GPIb/IX), and collagen (GPIa/IIa) are not correlated with an increased risk for stroke. *Stroke* 1997;**28**:1392–1395.
36. Corral J, Gonzalez-Conejero R, Rivera J, *et al.* HPA-1 genotype in arterial thrombosis — role of HPA-1b polymorphism in platelet function. *Blood Coagul Fibrinolysis* 1997;**8**:284–290.
37. Wagner KR, Giles WH, Johnson CJ, *et al.* Platelet glycoprotein receptor IIIa polymorphism P1A2 and ischemic stroke risk: the Stroke Prevention in Young Women Study. *Stroke* 1998;**29**:581–585.
38. Ridker PM, Hennekens CH, Schmitz C, *et al.* PIA1/A2 polymorphism of platelet glycoprotein IIIa and risks of myocardial infarction, stroke, and venous thrombosis. *Lancet* 1997;**349**:385–388.
39. Carter AM, Catto AJ, Bamford JM, *et al.* Platelet GP IIIa PlA and GP Ib variable number tandem repeat polymorphisms and markers of platelet activation in acute stroke. *Arterioscler Thromb Vasc Biol* 1998;**18**:1124–1131.
40. Carter AM, Ossei-Gerning N, Wilson IJ, *et al.* Association of the platelet Pl(A) polymorphism of glycoprotein IIb/IIIa and the fibrinogen Bbeta 448 polymorphism with myocardial infarction and extent of coronary artery disease. *Circulation* 1997;**96**:1424–1431.

41. Renner W, Winkler M, Hoffmann C, *et al.* The PlA1/A2 polymorphism of platelet glycoprotein IIIa is not associated with deep venous thrombosis. *Int Angiol* 2001;**20**:148–151.
42. Renner W, Brodmann M, Winkler M, *et al.* The PLA1/A2 polymorphism of platelet glycoprotein IIIa is not associated with peripheral arterial disease. *Thromb Haemost* 2001;**85**:745–746.
43. Goodall AH, Curzen N, Panesar M, *et al.* Increased binding of fibrinogen to glycoprotein IIIa-proline33 (HPA-1b, PlA2, Zwb) positive platelets in patients with cardiovascular disease. *Eur Heart J* 1999;**20**:742–747.
44. Feng D, Lindpaintner K, Larson MG, *et al.* Increased platelet aggregability associated with platelet GPIIIa PlA2 polymorphism: the Framingham Offspring Study. *Arterioscler Thromb Vasc Biol* 1999;**19**:1142–1147.
45. Meiklejohn DJ, Urbaniak SJ, Greaves M. Platelet glycoprotein IIIa polymorphism HPA 1b (PlA2): no association with platelet fibrinogen binding. *Br J Haematol* 1999;**105**:664–666.
46. Michelson AD, Furman MI, Goldschmidt-Clermont P, *et al.* Platelet GP IIIa Pl(A) polymorphisms display different sensitivities to agonists. *Circulation* 2000;**101**:1013–1018.
47. Bennett JS, Catella-Lawson F, Rut AR, *et al.* Effect of the Pl(A2) alloantigen on the function of beta(3)-integrins in platelets. *Blood* 2001;**97**:3093–3099.
48. Lasne D, Krenn M, Pingault V, *et al.* Interdonor variability of platelet response to thrombin receptor activation: influence of PlA2 polymorphism. *Br J Haematol* 1997;**99**:801–807.
49. Vijayan KV, Huang TC, Liu Y, *et al.* Shear stress augments the enhanced adhesive phenotype of cells expressing the Pro33 isoform of integrin beta3. *FEBS Lett* 2003;**540**:41–46.
50. Sajid M, Vijayan KV, Souza S, *et al.* PlA polymorphism of integrin beta3 differentially modulates cellular migration on extracellular matrix proteins. *Arterioscler Thromb Vasc Biol* 2002;**22**:1984–1989.
51. Vijayan KV, Liu Y, Sun W, *et al.* The Pro33 isoform of integrin beta3 enhances outside-in signaling in human platelets by regulating the activation of serine/threonine phosphatases. *J Biol Chem* 2005;**280**:21756–21762.
52. Goto S, Ikeda Y, Saldivar E, *et al.* Distinct mechanisms of platelet aggregation as a consequence of different shearing flow conditions. *J Clin Invest* 1998;**101**:479–486.
53. Goto S, Salomon DR, Ikeda Y, *et al.* Characterization of the unique mechanism mediating the shear-dependent binding of soluble von Willebrand factor to platelets. *J Biol Chem* 1995;**270**:23352–23361.

54. Lopez JA, Dong JF. Structure and function of the glycoprotein Ib-IX-V complex. *Curr Opin Hematol* 1997;**4**:323–329.
55. Kuijpers RW, Faber NM, Cuypers HT, *et al.* NH2-terminal globular domain of human platelet glycoprotein Ib alpha has a methionine 145/threonine145 amino acid polymorphism, which is associated with the HPA-2 (Ko) alloantigens. *J Clin Invest* 1992;**89**:381–384.
56. Jung SM, Plow EF, Moroi M. Polymorphism of platelet glycoprotein Ib in the United States. *Thromb Res* 1986;**42**:83–90.
57. Moroi M, Jung SM, Yoshida N. Genetic polymorphism of platelet glycoprotein Ib. *Blood* 1984;**64**:622–629.
58. Murata M, Matsubara Y, Kawano K, *et al.* Coronary artery disease and polymorphisms in a receptor mediating shear stress-dependent platelet activation. *Circulation* 1997;**96**:3281–3286.
59. Gonzalez-Conejero R, Lozano ML, Rivera J, *et al.* Polymorphisms of platelet membrane glycoprotein Ib associated with arterial thrombotic disease. *Blood* 1998;**92**:2771–2776.
60. Ito T, Ishida F, Shimodaira S, *et al.* Polymorphisms of platelet membrane glycoprotein Ib alpha and plasma von Willebrand factor antigen in coronary artery disease. *Int J Hematol* 1999;**70**:47–51.
61. Hato T, Minamoto Y, Fukuyama T, *et al.* Polymorphisms of HPA-1 through 6 on platelet membrane glycoprotein receptors are not a genetic risk factor for myocardial infarction in the Japanese population. *Am J Cardiol* 1997;**80**:1222–1224.
62. Ardissino D, Mannucci PM, Merlini PA, *et al.* Prothrombotic genetic risk factors in young survivors of myocardial infarction. *Blood* 1999;**94**:46–51.
63. Carter AM, Catto AJ, Bamford JM, *et al.* Platelet GP IIIa PlA and GP Ib variable number tandem repeat polymorphisms and markers of platelet activation in acute stroke. *Arterioscler Thromb Vasc Biol* 1998;**18**:1124–1131.
64. Li CQ, Garner SF, Davies J, *et al.* Threonine-145/methionine-145 variants of baculovirus produced recombinant ligand binding domain of GPIbalpha express HPA-2 epitopes and show equal binding of von Willebrand factor. *Blood* 2000;**95**:205–211.
65. Mazzucato M, Pradella P, de Angelis V, *et al.* Frequency and functional relevance of genetic threonine145/methionine145 dimorphism in platelet glycoprotein Ib alpha in an Italian population. *Transfusion* 1996;**36**:891–894.
66. Afshar-Kharghan V, Li CQ, Khoshnevis-Asl M, *et al.* Kozak sequence polymorphism of the glycoprotein (GP) Ibalpha gene is a major determinant of the plasma membrane levels of the platelet GP Ib-IX-V complex. *Blood* 1999;**94**:186–191.

67. Corral J, Lozano ML, Gonzalez-Conejero R, *et al.* A common polymorphism flanking the ATG initiator codon of GPIb alpha does not affect expression and is not a major risk factor for arterial thrombosis. *Thromb Haemost* 2000;**83**:23–28.
68. Kenny D, Muckian C, Fitzgerald DJ, *et al.* Platelet glycoprotein Ib alpha receptor polymorphisms and recurrent ischaemic events in acute coronary syndrome patients. *J Thromb Thrombolysis* 2002;**13**:13–19.
69. Croft SA, Hampton KK, Daly ME, *et al.* Kozak sequence polymorphism in the platelet GPIbalpha gene is not associated with risk of myocardial infarction. *Blood* 2000;**95**:2183–2184.
70. Clemetson KJ, Clemetson JM. Platelet collagen receptors. *Thromb Haemost* 2001;**86**:189–197.
71. Croft SA, Samani NJ, Teare MD, *et al.* Novel platelet membrane glycoprotein VI dimorphism is a risk factor for myocardial infarction. *Circulation* 2001;**104**:1459–1463.
72. Takagi S, Iwai N, Baba S, *et al.* A GPVI polymorphism is a risk factor for myocardial infarction in Japanese. *Atherosclerosis* 2002;**165**: 397–398.
73. Cole VJ, Staton JM, Eikelboom JW, *et al.* Collagen platelet receptor polymorphisms integrin alpha2beta1 C807T and GPVI Q317L and risk of ischemic stroke. *J Thromb Haemost* 2003;**1**:963–970.
74. Arepally G, McKenzie SE, Jiang XM, *et al.* Fc gamma RIIA H/R 131 polymorphism, subclass-specific IgG anti-heparin/platelet factor 4 antibodies and clinical course in patients with heparin-induced thrombocytopenia and thrombosis. *Blood* 1997;**89**:370–375.
75. Carlsson LE, Santoso S, Baurichter G, *et al.* Heparin-induced thrombocytopenia: new insights into the impact of the FcgammaRIIa-R-H131 polymorphism. *Blood* 1998;**92**:1526–1531.
76. Andre P, Delaney SM, LaRocca T, *et al.* P2Y12 regulates platelet adhesion/activation, thrombus growth, and thrombus stability in injured arteries. *J Clin Invest* 2003;**112**:398–406.
77. Takano S, Kimura J, Matsuoka I, *et al.* No requirement of P2X1 purinoceptors for platelet aggregation. *Eur J Pharmacol* 1999;**372**:305–309.
78. Foster CJ, Prosser DM, Agans JM, *et al.* Molecular identification and characterization of the platelet ADP receptor targeted by thienopyridine antithrombotic drugs. *J Clin Invest* 2001;**107**:1591–1598.
79. Fontana P, Dupont A, Gandrille S, *et al.* Adenosine diphosphate-induced platelet aggregation is associated with P2Y12 gene sequence variations in healthy subjects. *Circulation* 2003;**108**:989–995.

80. Hetherington SL, Singh RK, Lodwick D, *et al.* Dimorphism in the P2Y1 ADP receptor gene is associated with increased platelet activation response to ADP. *Arterioscler Thromb Vasc Biol* 2005;**25**:252–257.
81. Jefferson BK, Foster JH, McCarthy JJ, *et al.* Aspirin resistance and a single gene. *Am J Cardiol* 2005;**95**:805–808.
82. Greco NJ, Tonon G, Chen W, *et al.* Novel structurally altered P(2X1) receptor is preferentially activated by adenosine diphosphate in platelets and megakaryocytic cells. *Blood* 2001;**98**:100–107.
83. Weiss HJ, Turitto VT, Vicic WJ, *et al.* Effect of aspirin and dipyridamole on the interaction of human platelets with sub-endothelium: studies using citrated and native blood. *Thromb Haemost* 1981;**45**:136–141.
84. Final report on the aspirin component of the ongoing Physicians' Health Study. Steering Committee of the Physicians' Health Study Research Group. *N Engl J Med* 1989;**321**:129–135.
85. Thrombosis prevention trial: randomised trial of low-intensity oral anticoagulation with warfarin and low-dose aspirin in the primary prevention of ischaemic heart disease in men at increased risk. The Medical Research Council's General Practice Research Framework. *Lancet* 1998;**351**:233–241.
86. Gum PA, Kottke-Marchant K, Poggio ED, *et al.* Profile and prevalence of aspirin resistance in patients with cardiovascular disease. *Am J Cardiol* 2001;**88**:230–235.
87. Eikelboom JW, Hirsh J, Weitz JI, *et al.* Aspirin-resistant thromboxane biosynthesis and the risk of myocardial infarction, stroke, or cardiovascular death in patients at high risk for cardiovascular events. *Circulation* 2002;**105**:1650–1655.
88. Gum PA, Kottke-Marchant K, Welsh PA, *et al.* A prospective, blinded determination of the natural history of aspirin resistance among stable patients with cardiovascular disease. *J Am Coll Cardiol* 2003;**41**:961–965.
89. Mason PJ, Jacobs AK, Freedman JE. Aspirin resistance and atherothrombotic disease. *J Am Coll Cardiol* 2005;**46**:986–993.
90. Szczeklik A, Undas A, Sanak M, *et al.* Relationship between bleeding time, aspirin and the PlA1/A2 polymorphism of platelet glycoprotein IIIa. *Br J Haematol* 2000;**110**:965–967.
91. Undas A, Brummel K, Musial J, *et al.* Pl(A2) polymorphism of beta(3) integrins is associated with enhanced thrombin generation and impaired antithrombotic action of aspirin at the site of microvascular injury. *Circulation* 2001;**104**:2666–2672.
92. Walter DH, Schachinger V, Elsner M, *et al.* Platelet glycoprotein IIIa polymorphisms and risk of coronary stent thrombosis. *Lancet* 1997;**350**:1217–1219.

93. Kastrati A, Schomig A, Seyfarth M, *et al.* PlA polymorphism of platelet glycoprotein IIIa and risk of restenosis after coronary stent placement. *Circulation* 1999;**99**:1005–1010.
94. Kastrati A, Koch W, Gawaz M, *et al.* PlA polymorphism of glycoprotein IIIa and risk of adverse events after coronary stent placement. *J Am Coll Cardiol* 2000;**36**:84–89.
95. Lincoff AM, Califf RM, Topol EJ. Platelet glycoprotein IIb/IIIa receptor blockade in coronary artery disease. *J Am Coll Cardiol* 2000;**35**:1103–1115.
96. Rozalski M, Watala C. Antagonists of platelet fibrinogen receptor are less effective in carriers of Pl(A2) polymorphism of beta(3) integrin. *Eur J Pharmacol* 2002;**454**:1–8.
97. Weber AA, Jacobs C, Meila D, *et al.* No evidence for an influence of the human platelet antigen-1 polymorphism on the antiplatelet effects of glycoprotein IIb/IIIa inhibitors. *Pharmacogenetics* 2002;**12**:581–583.
98. O'Connor FF, Shields DC, Fitzgerald A, *et al.* Genetic variation in glycoprotein IIb/IIIa (GPIIb/IIIa) as a determinant of the responses to an oral GPIIb/IIIa antagonist in patients with unstable coronary syndromes. *Blood* 2001;**98**:3256–3260.
99. Cannon CP. Effectiveness of clopidogrel versus aspirin in preventing acute myocardial infarction in patients with symptomatic atherothrombosis (CAPRIE trial). *Am J Cardiol* 2002;**90**:760–762.
100. Mehta SR. Aspirin and clopidogrel in patients with ACS undergoing PCI: CURE and PCI-CURE. *J Invasive Cardiol* 2003;**15**(Suppl B): 17B–20B.
101. Gurbel PA, Bliden KP. Interpretation of platelet inhibition by clopidogrel and the effect of non-responders. *J Thromb Haemost* 2003;**1**:1318–1319.
102. Gurbel PA, Bliden KP, Hiatt BL, *et al.* Clopidogrel for coronary stenting: response variability, drug resistance, and the effect of pretreatment platelet reactivity. *Circulation* 2003;**107**:2908–2913.
103. Fontana P, Dupont A, Gandrille S, *et al.* Adenosine diphosphate-induced platelet aggregation is associated with P2Y12 gene sequence variations in healthy subjects. *Circulation* 2003;**108**:989–995.
104. Drachman JG, Jarvik GP, Mehaffey MG. Autosomal dominant thrombocytopenia: incomplete megakaryocyte differentiation and linkage to human chromosome 10. *Blood* 2000;**96**:118–125.
105. Mehaffey MG, Newton AL, Gandhi MJ, *et al.* X-linked thrombocytopenia caused by a novel mutation of GATA-1. *Blood* 2001;**98**:2681–2688.
106. Cheung CC, Martin IC, Zenger KR, *et al.* Quantitative trait loci for steady-state platelet count in mice. *Mamm Genome* 2004;**15**:784–797.

107. Evans DM, Zhu G, Duffy DL, *et al.* Multivariate QTL linkage analysis suggests a QTL for platelet count on chromosome 19q. *Eur J Hum Genet* 2004;**12**:835–842.
108. Garcia A, Zitzmann N, Watson SP. Analyzing the platelet proteome. *Semin Thromb Hemost* 2004;**30**:485–489.
109. http://ca.expasy.org/ch2d/.
110. Marcus K, Immler D, Sternberger J, *et al.* Identification of platelet proteins separated by two-dimensional gel electrophoresis and analyzed by matrix assisted laser desorption/ionization-time of flight-mass spectrometry and detection of tyrosine-phosphorylated proteins. *Electrophoresis* 2000;**21**:2622–2636.
111. Maguire PB, Fitzgerald DJ. Platelet proteomics. *J Thromb Haemost* 2003;**1**:1593–1601.
112. Maguire PB. Platelet proteomics: identification of potential therapeutic targets. *Pathophysiol Haemost Thromb* 2003;**33**:481–486.
113. Maguire PB, Moran N, Cagney G, *et al.* Application of proteomics to the study of platelet regulatory mechanisms. *Trends Cardiovasc Med* 2004;**14**:207–220.
114. Garcia A, Watson SP, Dwek RA, *et al.* Applying proteomics technology to platelet research. *Mass Spectrom Rev* 2005;**24**:918–930.
115. Perrotta PL, Bahou WF. Proteomics in platelet science. *Curr Hematol Rep* 2004;**3**:462–469.
116. Yates JR, III. Mass spectrometry. From genomics to proteomics. *Trends Genet* 2000;**16**:5–8.
117. Gravel P, Sanchez JC, Walzer C, *et al.* Human blood platelet protein map established by two-dimensional polyacrylamide gel electrophoresis. *Electrophoresis* 1995;**16**:1152–1159.
118. O'Neill EE, Brock CJ, von Kriegsheim AF, *et al.* Towards complete analysis of the platelet proteome. *Proteomics* 2002;**2**:288–305.
119. Garcia A, Prabhakar S, Brock CJ, *et al.* Extensive analysis of the human platelet proteome by two-dimensional gel electrophoresis and mass spectrometry. *Proteomics* 2004;**4**:656–668.
120. Garcia A, Prabhakar S, Hughan S, *et al.* Differential proteome analysis of TRAP-activated platelets: involvement of DOK-2 and phosphorylation of RGS proteins. *Blood* 2004;**103**:2088–2095.
121. Coppinger JA, Cagney G, Toomey S, *et al.* Characterization of the proteins released from activated platelets leads to localization of novel platelet proteins in human atherosclerotic lesions. *Blood* 2004;**103**:2096–2104.

122. Weyrich AS, Lindemann S, Tolley ND, *et al.* Change in protein phenotype without a nucleus: translational control in platelets. *Semin Thromb Hemost* 2004;**30**:491–498.
123. Weyrich AS, Zimmerman GA. Evaluating the relevance of the platelet transcriptome. *Blood* 2003;**102**:1550–1551.
124. Gnatenko DV, Dunn JJ, McCorkle SR, *et al.* Transcript profiling of human platelets using microarray and serial analysis of gene expression. *Blood* 2003;**101**:2285–2293.
125. Bahou WF, Gnatenko DV. Platelet transcriptome: the application of microarray analysis to platelets. *Semin Thromb Hemost* 2004;**30**:473–484.
126. Weyrich AS, Dixon DA, Pabla R, *et al.* Signal-dependent translation of a regulatory protein, Bcl-3, in activated human platelets. *Proc Natl Acad Sci USA* 1998;**95**:5556–5561.
127. Lindemann S, Tolley ND, Dixon DA, *et al.* Activated platelets mediatc inflammatory signaling by regulated interleukin 1beta synthesis. *J Cell Biol* 2001;**154**:485–490.
128. Roth GJ, Hickey MJ, Chung DW, *et al.* Circulating human blood platelets retain appreciable amounts of poly (A)+ RNA. *Biochem Biophys Res Commun* 1989;**160**:705–710.
129. Booyse FM, Rafelson ME, Jr. Studies on human platelets. I. Synthesis of platelet protein in a cell-free system. *Biochim Biophys Acta* 1968;**166**:689–697.
130. Belloc F, Hourdille P, Boisseau MR, *et al.* Protein synthesis in human platelets correlation with platelet size. *Nouv Rev Fr Hematol* 1982;**24**:369–373.
131. Nguyen YH, Mills AA, Stanbridge EJ. Assembly of the QM protein onto the 60S ribosomal subunit occurs in the cytoplasm. *J Cell Biochem* 1998;**68**:281–285.
132. Denis MM, Tolley ND, Bunting M, *et al.* Escaping the nuclear confines: signal-dependent pre-mRNA splicing in anucleate platelets. *Cell* 2005;**122**:379–391.
133. Macaulay IC, Carr P, Farrugia R, *et al.* Analysing the platelet transcriptome. *Vox Sang* 2004;**87**(Suppl 2):42–46.
134. Burge CB. Chipping away at the transcriptome. *Nat Genet* 2001;**27**:232–234.
135. Bertucci F, Houlgatte R, Benziane A, *et al.* Gene expression profiling of primary breast carcinomas using arrays of candidate genes. *Hum Mol Genet* 2000;**9**:2981–2991.
136. Golub TR, Slonim DK, Tamayo P, *et al.* Molecular classification of cancer: class discovery and class prediction by gene expression monitoring. *Science* 1999;**286**:531–537.

137. Alizadeh AA, Eisen MB, Davis RE, *et al.* Distinct types of diffuse large B-cell lymphoma identified by gene expression profiling. *Nature* 2000;**403**:503–511.
138. Tuteja R, Tuteja N. Serial analysis of gene expression (SAGE): application in cancer research. *Med Sci Monit.* 2004;**10**:RA132-RA140.
139. Tuteja R, Tuteja N. Serial analysis of gene expression (SAGE): unraveling the bioinformatics tools. *Bioessays* 2004;**26**:916–922.
140. Rox JM, Bugert P, Muller J, *et al.* Gene expression analysis in platelets from a single donor: evaluation of a PCR-based amplification technique. *Clin Chem* 2004;**50**:2271–2278.
141. Bugert P, Dugrillon A, Gunaydin A, *et al.* Messenger RNA profiling of human platelets by microarray hybridization. *Thromb Haemost* 2003;**90**:738–748.
142. McRedmond JP, Park SD, Reilly DF, *et al.* Integration of proteomics and genomics in platelets: a profile of platelet proteins and platelet-specific genes. *Mol Cell Proteomics* 2004;**3**:133–144.
143. Harvey PJ, Keightley AM, Lam YM, *et al.* A single nucleotide polymorphism at nucleotide-1793 in the von Willebrand factor (VWF) regulatory region is associated with plasma VWF:Ag levels. *Br J Haematol* 2000;**109**:349–353.
144. Dai K, Gao W, Ruan C. The Sma I polymorphism in the von Willebrand factor gene associated with acute ischemic stroke. *Thromb Res* 2001;**104**:389–395.
145. Listi F, Candore G, Lio D, *et al.* Association between platelet endothelial cellular adhesion molecule 1 (PECAM-1/CD31) polymorphisms and acute myocardial infarction: a study in patients from Sicily. *Eur J Immunogenet* 2004;**31**:175–178.
146. Fang L, Wei H, Chowdhury SH, *et al.* Association of Leu125Val polymorphism of platelet endothelial cell adhesion molecule-1 (PECAM-1) gene and soluble level of PECAM-1 with coronary artery disease in Asian Indians. *Indian J Med Res* 2005;**121**:92–99.
147. Elrayess MA, Webb KE, Bellingan GJ, *et al.* R643G polymorphism in PECAM-1 influences transendothelial migration of monocytes and is associated with progression of CHD and CHD events. *Atherosclerosis* 2004;**177**:127–135.
148. Klinkhardt U, Dragutinovic I, Harder S. P-selectin (CD62p) and P-selectin glycoprotein ligand-1 (PSGL-1) polymorphisms: minor phenotypic differences in the formation of platelet-leukocyte aggregates and response to clopidogrel. *Int J Clin Pharmacol Ther* 2005;**43**:255–263.
149. Herrmann SM, Ricard S, Nicaud V, *et al.* Polymorphisms in the genes encoding platelet-derived growth factor A and alpha receptor. *J Mol Med* 2000;**78**:287–292.

150. Kaye DM, Smirk B, Finch S, *et al.* Interaction between cardiac sympathetic drive and heart rate in heart failure: modulation by adrenergic receptor genotype. *J Am Coll Cardiol* 2004;**44**:2008–2015.
151. Busjahn A, Li GH, Faulhaber HD, *et al.* beta-2 adrenergic receptor gene variations, blood pressure, and heart size in normal twins. *Hypertension* 2000;**35**:555–560.
152. Belfer I, Buzas B, Evans C, *et al.* Haplotype structure of the beta adrenergic receptor genes in US Caucasians and African Americans. *Eur J Hum Genet* 2005;**13**:341–351.
153. Biggart S, Chin D, Fauchon M, *et al.* Association of genetic polymorphisms in the ACE, ApoE, and TGF beta genes with early onset ischemic heart disease. *Clin Cardiol* 1998;**21**:831–836.
154. Gourley IS, Denofrio D, Rand W, *et al.* The effect of recipient cytokine gene polymorphism on cardiac transplantation outcome. *Hum Immunol* 2004;**65**:248–254.
155. Aziz T, Hasleton P, Hann AW, *et al.* Transforming growth factor beta in relation to cardiac allograft vasculopathy after heart transplantation. *J Thorac Cardiovasc Surg* 2000;**119**:700–708.

7 Future Strategies for the Development of Antiplatelet Drugs

Robert A. Harrington

Introduction

In this chapter we will briefly discuss the central role that platelets play in the development of cardiovascular disease while recognizing that this topic is more completely explored in Chapter 1. Because of the platelet's central role in both the pathogenesis and the complications of cardiovascular disease, antiplatelet agents have emerged as a cornerstone therapy for patients with atherosclerotic vascular disease. We will discuss general issues and concepts of regulated drug development while looking at the field from the perspective of a clinician rather than focusing on regulatory requirements. In our specific focus on antiplatelet drug development, we will examine issues germane to both oral and parenteral drug preparations. Finally, we will review the various diseases for which antiplatelet therapies have proven clinical benefits and consider specific concepts and challenges relevant to those indications.

Arterial Thrombosis, Platelets, Cardiovascular Disease, and Antiplatelet Therapies

Following vascular injury, either induced, as with coronary intervention, or spontaneous, as with acute coronary syndromes, a complex series of interrelated events occurs that involves platelets and soluble coagulation proteins, resulting in the generation of thrombin, the formation of fibrin and, ultimately, a platelet-rich thrombus.[1] Platelet adhesion is critical to the initial response to any vascular injury, and the subsequent formation of the platelet aggregate provides the rich phospholipid surface necessary for the assembly of prothrombinase and the subsequent conversion of prothrombin to thrombin. So, while it is commonly taught and assumed that platelet hemostasis and coagulation are distinctly separate processes, they are in fact highly interrelated and dependent upon one another to provide maximal thrombotic response to vascular injury. The pivotal role of the platelet in these processes provides a strong biological rationale for antiplatelet therapy being a cornerstone therapy for a diverse group of vascular conditions.[2]

Currently aspirin, the ADP-receptor blocker clopidogrel, and the intravenous glycoprotein IIb/IIIa inhibitors are indicated in a variety of acute and chronic cardiovascular diseases (Table 1). These agents have all been shown to improve clinical outcomes in large-scale randomized controlled trials (RCTs), the gold standard for assessing therapeutic efficacy.

Aspirin is used in the treatment of all acute and chronic coronary syndromes. Its benefits are unquestioned; its safety is quite acceptable; and the cost-benefit ratio is extremely favorable.[3] Yet, even this universally-used antiplatelet therapy has limitations: its optimal dosing for both acute and chronic use is unknown; its antiplatelet effects are modest and confined to a single inhibitory pathway; some patients do not respond to its

Table 1. Commercially available antiplatelet therapies.

Agent	Usual delivery mode	Most common indications for use
Aspirin	Oral	STE AMI, NSTE ACS, PCI, CABG, CVA, TIA, secondary prevention, PAD, CVD, primary prevention
Clopidogrel	Oral	STE AMI, NSTE ACS, PCI, secondary prevention, PAD, CVD
Abciximab	Intravenous	PCI, including STE AMI
Eptifibatide	Intravenous	NSTE ACS, PCI
Tirofiban	Intravenous	NSTE ACS

STE AMI = ST-elevation acute myocardial infarction; NSTE ACS = non-ST-elevation acute coronary syndrome; PCI = percutaneous coronary intervention; CABG = coronary artery bypass graft surgery; CVA = cerebrovascular accident; TIA = transient ischemic attack; PAD = peripheral arterial disease; CVD = cerebrovascular disease.

measured antiplatelet effects ("aspirin resistance"); and some patients continue to have acute ischemic events despite ongoing aspirin therapy ("aspirin failures").

Likewise, clopidogrel has been proven beneficial in a number of acute and chronic cardiovascular indications. In these studies it has typically been shown to add incrementally to the positive effects of aspirin, but in one large study[4] it was shown to be marginally superior to aspirin in patients with chronic vascular disease. As with aspirin, clopidogrel therapy has limitations that include uncertainty about optimal dosing, questions about resistance, and issues regarding the lack of reversibility in situations where bleeding risks are high, as when patients with acute coronary syndromes require coronary artery bypass surgery. These limitations have led investigators to explore new modes of ADP blockade that will address some of these issues.

The intravenous glycoprotein (GP) IIb/IIIa inhibitors (abciximab, eptifibatide, and tirofiban) have been shown to reduce the ischemic complications of percutaneous coronary intervention (PCI)[5] and to reduce the risk of the composite of death and myocardial infarction among patients with non–ST-elevation acute coronary syndromes (NSTE ACS).[6] They have been used in combination with other platelet inhibitors, including both aspirin and clopidogrel, as well as with anticoagulants such as unfractionated heparin, low-molecular-weight heparin, and direct thrombin inhibitors (DTI). While the clinical value of these intravenous platelet blockers has been confirmed in a large number of RCTs, the long-term administration of oral GP IIb/IIIa inhibitors has not been shown to be effective, and may in fact carry an increased risk of mortality among treated patients.[7] Questions thus raised by the long experience with this class of antiplatelet therapy include how best to combine various antithrombotic therapies for maximal benefit while minimizing bleeding risk, and how best to assess acute versus more long-term effects of similar therapies.

Drug Development

Therapeutic drug development in the United States is regulated by the Food and Drug Administration.[8] Because of this, a number of rules and regulations must be adhered to in the process of evaluating a new therapeutic agent. In general, questions that should be addressed in the evaluation of any new therapeutic drug, biological agent, or device include: is the new therapy effective in improving clinical outcomes (do patients live longer, feel better, or avoid unpleasant experiences such as procedures)? Is the new therapy better than alternative (including standard) therapies? Is the new therapy safer than alternative therapies? What will or what does the new therapy cost? These basic questions set the framework for developing any new human therapeutic agent or device. They are essential for clinicians to consider before introducing new therapies into their clinical practice. They guide the regulators as they consider the value of a therapy being proposed for market approval. Increasingly, these questions are also being asked by payers, including the U.S. government, as measurements of quality in clinical care are increasingly linked to evidence-based guidelines and concepts such as pay-for-performance take hold.[9]

Understanding some basic principles of drug development is worthwhile for both the investigator considering the evaluation of new therapies as well as for the clinician who would like more insight into the process of this evaluation. Most drug development proceeds from discovery to preclinical evaluation to clinical testing. We will focus on the basics of clinical testing for new therapies.

Most cardiovascular drugs are evaluated first in Phase 1 studies involving normal human volunteers. These trials typically involve small numbers of subjects (usually a few dozen or fewer in the typical study), with the primary intent being to examine tolerability, gross safety effects, pharmacokinetics, and pharmacodynamics (PK/PD). Additional Phase 1 studies might study the effects of food on drug absorption, the interaction with other medications, or the PK/PD relationships in special groups (elderly, renally impaired, etc.). These studies are most frequently performed in dedicated Phase 1 units where there is close supervision. Understanding safety and some basic mechanistic issues with the drug are the goals of this development phase.

Phase 2 studies typically begin the process of introducing a new therapy into the ultimate patient groups of interest (i.e. those with coronary artery disease or those with heart failure). These studies are usually done in the health care setting (both inpatient and outpatient areas) with patients who have the relevant disease. Here, the goal is to expand upon the safety evaluation that began in the Phase 1 studies by extending those observations into a group of patients who have the actual disease, take the usual medications for the disease, and exhibit other comorbidities that might ultimately affect how the new therapy works or will be used in actual practice. Phase 2 trials typically involve hundreds, and occasionally a few thousands, of patients. The primary focus is still on safety and on understanding the adverse effects of a potential therapy in a higher-risk group of patients than the normal volunteers who were exposed to the therapy in Phase 1 studies. Understanding PK/PD relationships is often critical in these studies, as is the delineation of whether or not the drug actually has the intended biological effect in the clinical setting. To accomplish this last goal, Phase 2 trials typically rely upon measurement of a variety of biomarkers to try to establish that the therapy has the potential to improve clinical outcomes. Perhaps one of the best examples of this is in the testing of new antithrombotic regimens for the treatment of ST-elevation acute myocardial infarction. In many of these Phase 2 studies the primary efficacy measure is either the use of acute angiography to measure coronary blood flow (TIMI flow)[10] or the use of static and dynamic ECGs to assess the speed and completeness of ST-segment resolution.[11] Clinical outcomes are usually measured in these studies and may be suggestive of a drug effect; however, most times the typical Phase 2 study lacks adequate statistical power to demonstrate an effect of the new therapy on important clinical outcomes (i.e. death, myocardial infarction, need for procedures, rehospitalization).

Phase 3 studies are the large, definitive studies of efficacy and safety. These trials typically involve hundreds to many thousands of patients. The number of patients is determined by the risk within the population (the anticipated event rate) and the anticipated effect of the new therapy relative to the control therapy (either placebo or an active comparator). Smaller estimated effects of the therapy require larger sample sizes to increase the likelihood of detecting that effect, if it truly exists. (Clinicians interested in Phase 3 drug development should familiarize themselves with basic statistical concepts such as Type 1 and 2 errors as well as power.) These studies usually aim to determine if a new therapy has incremental benefit compared with the current standards. As such, meaningful clinical events either alone (such as death) or in some composite (death,

MI, or revascularization) are the primary measure of interest in Phase 3 studies. The large sample size also typically provides a reliable estimate of important side effects of the treatment, such as bleeding. Regulatory approval of a new drug for cardiovascular use typically requires at least two Phase 3 studies with positive findings, though a single large trial with definitive endpoints (such as mortality) and convincing results might be acceptable.

Thus one can see that the process of developing a new cardiovascular therapeutic is complex, time-consuming, and resource-intensive. The entire process from the start of Phase 1 through the process of applying for new drug approval typically takes many years and a large amount of capital investment.[12] Yet, even after the drug is appropriately approved for market use, typically many questions remain as to the optimal way for clinicians to use the medication in practice. Frequently, therefore, a number of additional Phase 3 (new indications) and Phase 4 (extension of prior knowledge) trials are performed to provide the clinical community with answers regarding the agent's use in special populations (the advanced elderly, children, those with renal failure, etc.), in new dosing strategies, or in combination with other therapies.

Antiplatelet Drug Development

Now we will consider some of the key issues and considerations specific to the development of antiplatelet therapies for use in the prevention and treatment of cardiovascular diseases. Table 2 lists the common cardiovascular indications for which antiplatelet drug therapies have proven value. Understanding some of the key concepts surrounding their use in these indications allows us to consider how best to approach future antiplatelet drug development.

The challenges in antiplatelet drug development fall into three categories. The first challenge has to do with the clinical indication, acute or chronic, which determines whether the drug is to be delivered as an intravenous agent or in oral form. The second challenge includes a number of general considerations that we will detail below. The final challenge is the special circumstances associated with the individual disease state.

Table 2. Clinical settings in which to consider use of antiplatelet therapies.

Acute coronary syndromes (ACS)

- ST-elevation myocardial infarction (STEMI)
- Non-ST-elevation acute myocardial infarction (NSTEMI)
- Unstable angina (UA)

Coronary revascularization

- Percutaneous coronary intervention (PCI)
- Coronary artery bypass graft surgery (CABG)

Acute cerebrovascular accident (CVA) or transient ischemic attack (TIA)
Acute peripheral occlusion
Secondary prevention

- Coronary artery disease (CAD)/acute coronary syndrome (ACS)
- CVA/TIA
- Peripheral arterial disease (PAD)

Congestive heart failure
Atrial fibrillation
Mechanical heart valves

Adapted from: Table 2. Thrombosis-dependent acute and chronic cardiovascular disease. In: Harrington RA. Developing drugs to prevent and treat arterial thrombosis. *Cardiol Rounds* 2003;**7**(7). Used by permission.

Acute versus chronic usage and advantages/limitations of IV versus oral preparations

There are advantages and disadvantages to drugs being available only as intravenous preparations. Typically, intravenous preparations are used in the acute care setting where the rapid onset of effect is considered critical to its benefit. These agents usually have more predictable pharmacokinetic (and consequently pharmacodynamic) profiles since they are not dependent on gastrointestinal absorption, which may be abnormal in settings of acute illness, including with hemodynamic instability. The effects of these agents frequently can be rapidly terminated with cessation of the infusion. This might be valuable at the end of an anticipated course of therapy, for example a percutaneous coronary intervention, or when a complication such as serious bleeding occurs. Finally, in the acute care setting, elderly cardiovascular patients frequently have concomitant gastrointestinal symptoms, including nausea and vomiting, that prohibit or limit the reliability of oral drug delivery.

Intravenous antiplatelet therapies have limitations as well. Given the requirements for delivery, their use is confined to the acute care setting. There is obviously a greater degree of sophistication of the health care system required in this setting since the use of intravenous medications requires venous access, perhaps special storage of the product, special handling and preparation, and the necessary delivery equipment, including IV pumps.

The ability to deliver antiplatelet therapies in an oral form overcomes most of these limitations and makes it attractive to use the therapy in a wide variety of health care settings, thereby allowing the broadest number of patients to benefit from effective therapies. From a public health perspective, this is a desirable characteristic given the global burden of cardiovascular disease. However, the advantages of intravenous therapy become the limitations of oral therapies. Particularly critical is obtaining an adequate understanding of the PK/PD relationships of oral drugs among the patient populations who will ultimately be treated with the agents. Having knowledge of how rapidly the drugs work, interpatient variability in response, and key predictors of biological effect are critical precursors to designing an appropriate Phase 3 program that will test the clinical effectiveness of the drug.

General issues to consider in antiplatelet drug development

There are a number of questions to consider as one works through how best to develop an antiplatelet drug for use in cardiovascular disease. Is this a disease state that necessitates very rapid and predictably sustained platelet inhibition? Is there an ability to assay the biological effect of the therapy? Is this felt to be necessary and/or desirable? Is there an understanding of the relationships between the drug's pharmacokinetics and its pharmacodynamic effects? Does this agent interact, either kinetically or dynamically, with other antithrombotic drugs? Is there an intention to provide this platelet inhibitor as monotherapy or in combination with other antithrombotic therapies? As an extension of that, is it possible or even desirable to perform placebo-controlled studies, or does the clinical setting necessitate that any comparison with standard therapy include an active comparator? Will the drug be administered only in the acute setting or is it anticipated that it will be beneficial in the chronic setting as well? What are the issues that might predict whether or not a therapy effective acutely is also effective in the more chronic clinical setting?

Developing antiplatelet therapies for use in patients with NSTE ACS and during PCI

Most patients who present with NSTE ACS in the United States, and in many non-U.S. countries as well, undergo early cardiac catheterization and coronary-anatomy-driven revascularization due to data suggesting the superiority of invasive management over a more conservative approach.[13] Because of the high use of PCI revascularization among these NSTE ACS patients,[14] it is worthwhile considering antithrombotic drug development in general, and antiplatelet therapy specifically, for use during NSTE ACS

Table 3. Challenges in antiplatelet drug development.

Acute coronary syndromes

- Older population; increased comorbidities
- United States-based practice
  - Early catheterization/PCI/CABG
  - Pressures on hospital length of stay
- Multiple effective drugs already in use
- Monitoring effects (assays and interpretation)

Percutaneous coronary intervention

- "Upstream" ACS treatment
- Multiple effective drugs in lab
- Device-drug interactions
- Monitoring effects

ACS = Acute coronary syndrome(s); CABG = coronary artery bypass graft; PCI = percutaneous coronary intervention.
Adapted from: Table 3. Considerations and challenges in antithrombotic drug development for PCI and ACS. In: Harrington RA. Developing drugs to prevent and treat arterial thrombosis. *Cardiol Rounds* 2003;**7**(7). Used by permission.

and PCI as a continuation of a common indication since there is much in common between these two clinical situations that should be considered in the development process. Table 3 outlines some things to consider in each of the specific indications.

First, among the group of patients presenting with a NSTE ACS, one must consider the older age of the typical patient and a large number of both cardiovascular and non-cardiac comorbidities that make use of any drug, especially antithrombotic drugs, challenging. As one weighs the balance between potential antiplatelet therapy benefits and risks (especially bleeding), things such as renal insufficiency, history of stroke, and frailty should be considered before deciding upon treatment, and, ultimately, upon dosing strategies and combinations of therapies.[15] The complexities associated with dosing drugs in this group of patients should cause investigators to consider the benefits of including patients with high levels of comorbidity in the pivotal studies instead of excluding them, as is frequently done.[16]

The likelihood of early (< 48 hours) cardiac catheterization means that any drug strategy used at the time of acute presentation needs to be adequately studied in the setting of the cath lab as well. This is challenging when there are multiple effective therapies in this setting, as a key issue becomes how best to assess the value of the newer therapies. Do new therapies get added to standard therapies in an attempt to look for incremental benefit over current care, or do investigators examine new versus alternative strategies of antithrombotic care in an attempt to replace previous therapies? These considerations have implications for clinical trial design. For example, in the first situation, one might be able to test the new therapy against placebo in a conventional double-blind, placebo-controlled RCT. Perhaps one of the best examples of this is the development of both the platelet GP IIb/IIIa inhibitors for use among patients presenting with NSTE ACS.[6,17] Finally, in the NSTE ACS setting, rapidity of treatment is often considered essential since the risk of an adverse ischemic event is highest soon after the initial presentation and then declines over the ensuing days to weeks. Because of this, assuring that the antiplatelet effect is maximal may be important. There is controversy on this topic, mainly about how best to ascertain the optimal level of therapy.

Most drug development with antiplatelet agents has purposefully stayed away from requiring some assessment of platelet inhibition as a key element of guiding treatment. This has been true with both the GP IIb/IIIa inhibitors and clopidogrel. Early Phase 2 studies with various GP IIb/IIIa inhibitors delineated the relationship among drug dosing, drug levels, and an antiplatelet effect as determined by standard light transmittance aggregometry.[18] But no large Phase 3 study with these drugs in either NSTE ACS or PCI definitively established a firm relationship between either drug levels or effect and clinical outcomes; however, there is some data suggestive of a relationship between antiplatelet effect as measured by a point-of-care testing device and clinical outcome.[19] While not definitive, these data provide insight into the question of how much platelet inhibition is needed to provide a clinical benefit with various drugs. With the GP IIb/IIIa inhibitors, the GOLD study suggests that very high levels of a measured antiplatelet effect ($> 95\%$ ADP-induced aggregation inhibition) are required to achieve maximal clinical benefit.

Early Phase 2 studies with clopidogrel were limited in scope and the large Phase 3 trials were conducted without any reliance on secondary outcomes that would attempt to establish a relationship between drug antiplatelet effects and clinical outcome. Clopidogrel proved highly effective in a variety of clinical settings with a relatively modest measured antiplatelet effect. As newer ADP blockers were discovered and pushed forward in the development process, they were compared with clopidogrel. These studies frequently demonstrated that clopidogrel had a decent amount of interpatient variability in its antiplatelet effects and that the extent of ADP-measured aggregation inhibition was modest.[20] Additionally, the concept of "clopidogrel resistance" began to emerge, modeled after aspirin resistance.[21–23] Resistance has been defined as having limited response to the standard measures of platelet aggregation inhibition. But the critical question is whether or not this is really an important clinical entity with clopidogrel. In the recent COMMIT[24] study of clopidogrel compared with placebo in acute STEMI, clopidogrel exerts a mortality benefit in the first few days after randomization despite being given in a dosing strategy (no bolus or loading dose followed by 75 mg/day) that has little measured antiplatelet effect.

While understanding the relationships among dosing, drug concentrations (especially among target patient populations), and some measured biological effect (such as inhibition of platelet aggregation) is critical in early Phase 1 and 2 development, most investigators do not adequately study this in the large clinical outcome studies. It is challenging and operationally cumbersome to do so, and many industry representatives do not want their product to be tied to a measurement assay if it can be avoided during future use. But much could be learned by having some data that would establish the critical level of platelet inhibition required to achieve a clinical effect.

Percutaneous coronary intervention carries an obligatory need for antithrombotic therapy.[25] Because the PCI setting is an excellent model of atherosclerotic plaque rupture with subsequent risk of thrombosis and its potential ischemic complications, this has become a "proving ground" for the testing of a number of antithrombotic therapies. PCI has several favorable characteristics to guide the development of antithrombotic therapies: the patient population is large and with a spectrum of risk and comorbidities, the timing of the plaque disruption is well categorized, blood samples are easily obtained, and the presence of arterial access serves as a stimulus of bleeding allowing a concomitant assessment of risk.

But developing antiplatelet therapies in the PCI setting carries some of the same challenges as the NSTE ACS setting. Multiple effective antithrombotic drugs are being used in the catheterization laboratory to reduce the risk of ischemic complications during PCI. These include aspirin, heparin(s), GP IIb/IIIa inhibitors, clopidogrel, and direct thrombin inhibitors. Consequently, clinical studies of new antiplatelet therapies in PCI may involve placebo-controlled methods looking for modest incremental benefits of a new therapy or active control therapies looking to replace other therapies. These would include the testing of new strategies that may provide similar anti-ischemic effects but offer improved ease of use[26] or increased safety[27] over contemporary therapeutic strategies.[28] Likewise, defining whether or not a therapy's effects can or must be monitored before PCI is a critical question that is best answered prior to performing the definitive studies, but oftentimes is not known for many years following approval and marketing of the therapeutic agent.

In PCI, there is an agreed-upon minimum threshold of anticoagulation that must be achieved with unfractionated heparin to provide the best balance between efficacy and safety;[29,30] however, there is less agreement with the notion of monitoring antiplatelet effects. Retrospective analyses suggest that there is greater clinical effect when clopidogrel is given as a loading dose some number of hours prior to the procedure. The debate over the timing and the amount of a clopidogrel loading dose is steeped in the question of how rapidly and how high a level of inhibition can be achieved.[31]

In deciding how best to treat the PCI patient with antiplatelet therapy, investigators and treating clinicians need to consider any "upstream" therapy that was started acutely after the diagnosis of NSTE ACS was made. Patients will arrive in the lab with a variety of drugs "on board." How best to consider the addition of or replacement with other drugs requires knowledge of the upstream therapies. A good example of the complexities surrounding all of this might be the use of GP IIb/IIIa inhibitors among patients with NSTE ACS.[32]

Developing antiplatelet therapies for use in patients with STEMI

While NSTE ACS and STE acute myocardial infarction (AMI) share some common elements, the development of antiplatelet therapies for treating patients with STE AMI requires that different issues be considered beyond those discussed above in the setting of NSTE ACS. First, since there are two different reperfusion strategies in wide clinical use for the acute treatment of STE AMI, investigators need to consider whether a new antiplatelet therapy will be tested in the setting of primary PCI or in combination with fibrinolytic therapy. Additionally, each of these treatment strategies employs a variety of other antithrombotic drugs as integral parts of the acute therapy. In the setting of planned primary PCI, these other therapies include both anticoagulants as well as several antiplatelet agents such as aspirin, clopidogrel, and GP IIb/IIIa inhibitors. When developing an antiplatelet agent to be given with fibrinolytic therapy, it is important to consider other antithrombotics, but serious attention must be given to being able to delineate the incremental risk of intracranial hemorrhage beyond that observed with current therapy, especially considering the elderly population, who already have an increased risk of intracranial hemorrhage (ICH).[33,34]

There are some definitive advantages to testing the effects of an antiplatelet therapy as an acute reperfusion strategy. The platelet is a proven therapeutic target in this areas, with clinical outcomes benefits established for aspirin, clopidogrel, and abciximab.[2,24,35,36] The methodologies of Phase 2 studies using either acute or delayed angiographic, nuclear imaging, and electrocardiographic parameters as potential markers of meaningful clinical benefits are well established. Newer imaging modalities such as MRI are promising ways to measure even relatively small infarcts and potentially allow discrimination of modest effects of a novel treatment. The challenges include the large number of patients required to establish an accurate assessment of ICH risk and the sample sizes required to definitely ascertain a clinical benefit, which is commonly defined as an effect on mortality.

Developing antiplatelet therapies for use in patients with chronic coronary artery disease

There are some additional and unique challenges to consider when developing an antiplatelet therapy for long-term use. First, outside of the setting of an acute ischemic event, clinical event rates over time are relatively modest in a chronic coronary artery disease population, requiring investigators to consider designing studies that preferentially target higher-risk populations (for example, those with a recent acute ischemic event or those with multiple cardiac risk factors and/or associated comorbidities), enroll large samples, or have prolonged durations of follow-up. Each of these approaches has benefits and limitations. High-risk populations typically also have high-risk features for adverse drug effects, including serious bleeding. Balancing the potential for benefit against the risk of therapy among a group with extensive comorbid conditions, such as renal insufficiency and advanced age, can be complex and difficult.

Risk of bleeding is especially problematic in the chronic setting, since patients are much less likely to tolerate even minor bleeding events outside of the acute, life-threatening situation of ACS. One also needs to be concerned about issues such as drug compliance and reversibility, since patients will skip doses and will have procedures whereby they would prefer to stop taking an experimental antiplatelet agent. The difference in clinical effect when drugs are administered acutely versus when they are given chronically raises these issues as well. Perhaps one of the best examples of this is the difference in clinical effect observed with the intravenous GP IIb/IIIa inhibitors compared with the increased risk of mortality observed in the overview of the oral agents in the same class of drugs.[7]

Future Directions

Two oral antiplatelet therapies, aspirin and clopidogrel, as well as three intravenous glycoprotein inhibitors have a proven role in the management of patients with ischemic heart disease. However, as discussed above, there are a number of limitations of these agents, including their combinations and their dosing, which makes the search for new antiplatelet strategies an important one.

In addition to the imperative to better understand the use of currently available antiplatelet drugs, there are multiple ways to interfere with platelet function. New targets for potential therapeutic agents include the platelet thrombin receptor, other glycoprotein receptors, and ways to consider inhibiting platelet adhesion and activation. All these other targets provide a conceptual basis for developing new therapies, but their potential benefits must be established and quantified in appropriately designed RCTs.

References

1. Tolleson TR, Harrington RA, Topol EJ. Adjunctive therapies in coronary interventions. In: Serruys PW, Leon MD, Colombo A, Kutryk JB (eds.) *Textbook of Coronary Disease*. Martin Dunitz Publishing, 2000.
2. Antiplatelet Trialists' Collaboration. Collaborative overview of randomised trials of antiplatelet therapy. *BMJ* 1994;**308**:81–246.
3. Awtry EH, Loscalzo J. Aspirin. *Circulation* 2000;**101**:1206–1218.
4. CAPRIE Steering Committee. A randomised, blinded, trial of clopidogrel versus aspirin in patients at risk of ischaemic events (CAPRIE). *Lancet* 1996;**348**:1329–1339.
5. Kong DF, Hasselblad V, Harrington RA, White HD, Tcheng JE, Kandzari DE, Topol EJ, Califf RM. Meta-analysis of survival with platelet glycoprotein IIb/IIIa antagonists for percutaneous coronary interventions. *Am J Cardiol* 2003;**92**:651–655.
6. Boersma E, Harrington RA, Moliterno DJ, White H, Theroux P, Van de Werf F, de Torbal A, Armstrong PW, Wallentin LC, Wilcox RG, Simes J, Califf RM, Topol EJ, Simoons ML. Platelet glycoprotein IIb/IIIa inhibitors in acute coronary syndromes: a meta-analysis of all major randomised clinical trials. *Lancet* 2002;**359**:189–198. Erratum in: *Lancet* 2002;**359**(9323):2120.

7. Newby LK, Califf RM, White HD, Harrington RA, Van de Werf F, Granger CB, Simes RJ, Hasselblad V, Armstrong PW. The failure of orally administered glycoprotein IIb/IIIa inhibitors to prevent recurrent cardiac events. *Am J Med* 2002;**112**:647–658.
8. FDA Center for Drug Evaluation and Research resources page. Food and Drug Administration website. Available at: http://www.fda.gov/cder/index.html. Accessed January 26, 2006.
9. Centers for Medicare and Medicaid Services resources page. Department of Health and Human Services website. Available at http://www.cms.hhs.gov.
10. Giugliano RP, Roe MT, Harrington RA, Gibson CM, Zeymer U, Van de Werf F, Baran KW, Hobbach HP, Woodlief LH, Hannan KL, Greenberg S, Miller J, Kitt MM, Strony J, McCabe CH, Braunwald E, Califf RM; INTEGRITI Investigators. Combination reperfusion therapy with eptifibatide and reduced-dose tenecteplase for ST-elevation myocardial infarction: results of the integrilin and tenecteplase in acute myocardial infarction (INTEGRITI) Phase II Angiographic Trial. *J Am Coll Cardiol* 2003;**41**:1251–1260.
11. Krucoff MW, Johanson P, Baeza R, Crater SW, Dellborg M. Clinical utility of serial and continuous ST-segment recovery assessment in patients with acute ST-elevation myocardial infarction: assessing the dynamics of epicardial and myocardial reperfusion. *Circulation* 2004;**110**:e533–e539.
12. DiMasi JA, Hansen RW, Grabowski HG. The price of innovation: new estimates of drug development costs. *J Health Econ* 2003;**22**:151–185.
13. Mehta SR, Cannon CP, Fox KA, Wallentin L, Boden WE, Spacek R, Widimsky P, McCullough PA, Hunt D, Braunwald E, Yusuf S. Routine versus selective invasive strategies in patients with acute coronary syndromes: a collaborative meta-analysis of randomized trials. *JAMA* 2005;**293**:2908–2917.
14. Bhatt DL, Roe MT, Peterson ED, Li Y, Chen AY, Harrington RA, Greenbaum AB, Berger PB, Cannon CP, Cohen DJ, Gibson CM, Saucedo JF, Kleiman NS, Hochman JS, Boden WE, Brindis RG, Peacock WF, Smith SC Jr, Pollack CV Jr, Gibler WB, Ohman EM; CRUSADE Investigators. Utilization of early invasive management strategies for high-risk patients with non-ST-segment elevation acute coronary syndromes: results from the CRUSADE Quality Improvement Initiative. *JAMA* 2004;**292**:2096–2104.
15. Alexander KP, Chen AY, Roe MT, Newby LK, Gibson CM, Allen-LaPointe NM, Pollack C, Gibler WB, Ohman EM, Peterson ED; CRUSADE Investigators. Excess dosing of antiplatelet and antithrombin agents in the treatment of non-ST-segment elevation acute coronary syndromes. *JAMA* 2005;**294**:3108–3116.

16. Lee PY, Alexander KP, Hammill BG, Pasquali SK, Peterson ED. Representation of elderly persons and women in published randomized trials of acute coronary syndromes. *JAMA* 2001;**286**:708–713.
17. Yusuf S, Zhao F, Mehta SR, Chrolavicius S, Tognoni G, Fox KK. Clopidogrel in Unstable Angina to Prevent Recurrent Events Trial Investigators. Effects of clopidogrel in addition to aspirin in patients with acute coronary syndromes without ST-segment elevation. *N Engl J Med* 2001;**345**:494–502.
18. Berkowitz SD, Frelinger AL 3rd, Hillman RS. Progress in point-of-care laboratory testing for assessing platelet function. *Am Heart J* 1998;**136**(4 Pt 2 Suppl):S51–S65.
19. Steinhubl SR, Talley JD, Braden GA, Tcheng JE, Casterella PJ, Moliterno DJ, Navetta FI, Berger PB, Popma JJ, Dangas G, Gallo R, Sane DC, Saucedo JF, Jia G, Lincoff AM, Theroux P, Holmes DR, Teirstein PS, Kereiakes DJ. Point-of-care measured platelet inhibition correlates with a reduced risk of an adverse cardiac event after percutaneous coronary intervention: results of the GOLD (AU-Assessing Ultegra) multicenter study. *Circulation* 2001;**103**:2572–2578.
20. Gurbel PA, Bliden KP, Hiatt BL, O'Connor CM. Clopidogrel for coronary stenting response variability, drug resistance, and the effect of pretreatment platelet reactivity. *Circulation* 2003;**107**:2908–2913.
21. Gurbel PA, Bliden KP, Hayes KM, Yoho JA, Herzog WR, Tantry US. The relation of dosing to clopidogrel responsiveness and the incidence of high post-treatment platelet aggregation in patients undergoing coronary stenting. *J Am Coll Cardiol* 2005;**45**:1392–1396.
22. Matetzky S, Shenkman B, Guetta V, Shechter M, Bienart R, Goldenberg I, Novikov I, Pres H, Savion N, Varon D, Hod H. Clopidogrel resistance is associated with increased risk of recurrent atherothrombotic events in patients with acute myocardial infarction. *Circulation* 2004;**109**:3171–3175.
23. Gurbel PA, Bliden KP. Durability of platelet inhibition by clopidogrel. *Am J Cardiol* 2003;**91**:1123–1125.
24. Chen ZM, Jiang LX, Chen YP, Xie JX, Pan HC, Peto R, Collins R, Liu LS; COMMIT (ClOpidogrel and Metoprolol in Myocardial Infarction Trial) collaborative group. Addition of clopidogrel to aspirin in 45,852 patients with acute myocardial infarction: randomised placebo-controlled trial. *Lancet* 2005;**366**:1607–1621.
25. Popma JJ, Berger P, Ohman EM, Harrington RA, Grines C, Weitz JI. Antithrombotic therapy during percutaneous coronary intervention: the Seventh ACCP Conference on Antithrombotic and Thrombolytic Therapy. *Chest* 2004;**126**(3 Suppl):576S–599S.

26. Montalescot G, White HD, Gallo R, Cohen M, Stey PG, Aylward PE, Bode C, Chiariello M, King SB 3rd, Harrington RA, Desmet WJ, Macaya C, Steinhubl SR; STEEPLE Investigators. Enoxaparin versus unfractionated heparin in elective percutaneous coronary intervention. *N Engl J Med* 2006;**355**:1006–1017.
27. Lincoff AM, Kleiman NS, Kereiakes DJ, Feit F, Bittl JA, Jackman JD, Sarembock IJ, Cohen DJ, Spriggs D, Ebrahimi R, Keren G, Carr J, Cohen EA, Betriu A, Desmet W, Rutsch W, Wilcox RG, de Feyter PJ, Vahanian A, Topol EJ; REPLACE-2 Investigators. Long-term efficacy of bivalirudin and provisional glycoprotein IIb/IIIa blockade versus heparin and planned glycoprotein IIb/IIIa blockade during percutaneous coronary revascularization: REPLACE-2 randomized trial. *JAMA* 2004;**292**(6):696–703.
28. Siegel JP. Equivalence and noninferiority trials. *Am Heart J* 2000;**139**:S166–S170.
29. Brener SJ, Bhatt DL, Moliterno DJ, Schneider JP, Ellis SG, Topol EJ. Revisiting optimal anticoagulation with unfractionated heparin during coronary stent implantation. *Am J Cardiol* 2003;**92**:1468–1471.
30. Brener SJ, Moliterno DJ, Lincoff AM, Steinhubl SR, Wolski KE, Topol EJ. Relationship between activated clotting time and ischemic or hemorrhagic complications: analysis of four recent randomized clinical trials of percutaneous coronary intervention. *Circulation* 2004;**110**:994–998.
31. Tricoci P, Harrington RA, Valgimigli M. Letter regarding article by Patti *et al.*, "Randomized trial of high loading dose of clopidogrel for reduction of periprocedural myocardial infarction in patients undergoing coronary intervention: results from the ARMYDA-2 (Antiplatelet therapy for Reduction of MYocardial Damage during Angioplasty) study." *Circulation* 2005;**112**:e282; author reply e283.
32. Pieper KS, Tsiatis AA, Davidian M, Hasselblad V, Kleiman NS, Boersma E, Chang WC, Griffin J, Armstrong PW, Califf RM, Harrington RA. Differential treatment benefit of platelet glycoprotein IIb/IIIa inhibition with percutaneous coronary intervention versus medical therapy for acute coronary syndromes: exploration of methods. *Circulation* 2004;**109**:641–646.
33. Brener SJ, Lincoff AM, Bates ER, Jia G, Armstrong PW, Guetta V, Hochman JS, Savonitto S, Wilcox RG, White HD, Topol EJ; GUSTO V Investigators. The relationship between baseline risk and mortality in ST-elevation acute myocardial infarction treated with pharmacological reperfusion: insights from the Global Utilization of Strategies To open Occluded arteries (GUSTO) V trial. *Am Heart J* 2005;**150**:89–93.

34. Curtis JP, Alexander JH, Huang Y, Wallentin L, Verheugt FW, Armstrong PW, Krumholz HM, Van de Werf F, Danays T, Cheeks M, Granger CB; ASSENT-2 and ASSENT-3 Investigators. Efficacy and safety of two unfractionated heparin dosing strategies with tenecteplase in acute myocardial infarction (results from Assessment of the Safety and Efficacy of a New Thrombolytic Regimens 2 and 3). *Am J Cardiol* 2004;**94**:279–283.
35. Sabatine MS, Cannon CP, Gibson CM, Lopez-Sendon JL, Montalescot G, Theroux P, Lewis BS, Murphy SA, McCabe CH, Braunwald E; Clopidogrel as Adjunctive Reperfusion Therapy (CLARITY)-Thrombolysis in Myocardial Infarction (TIMI) 28 Investigators. Effect of clopidogrel pretreatment before percutaneous coronary intervention in patients with ST-elevation myocardial infarction treated with fibrinolytics: the PCI-CLARITY study. *JAMA* 2005;**294**:1224–1232.
36. Montalescot G, Borentain M, Payot L, Collet JP, Thomas D. Early versus late administration of glycoprotein IIb/IIIa inhibitors in primary percutaneous coronary intervention of acute ST-segment elevation myocardial infarction: a meta-analysis. *JAMA* 2004;**292**:362–366.

Index